30 Days to No More

Premenstrual Syndrome

A Doctors Proven Nutritional Program

by

Allen L. Lawrence, M.A., M.D., Ph.D.

and

Lisa Lawrence, M.S., Ph.D.

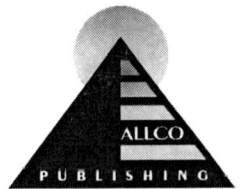

Tarzana, California

30 Days To No More PMS

ALLCO Publishing
18653 Ventura Blvd., Suite 384
Tarzana, CA 91356

Questions@30DaysNoMorePMS.com

About the Authors

ALLEN L. LAWRENCE, M.S., M.D., PH.D.

Allen Lawrence received his Medical degree from the University of California, California College of Medicine in Irvine, California. Dr. Allen Lawrence interned at University of Southern California's Los Angeles County General Hospital. He completed a residency in Obstetrics and Gynecology at Cedars Sinai Medical Center in Los Angeles, California. Dr. Lawrence obtained a Master's in Nutrition and a Ph.D. in Psychology at the Pacific Institute for Advanced Studies.

He has done extensive work and research in the area of women's medicine, stress and pain management, alternative healing, spiritual healing, nutrition and stress-related disorders.

Dr. Lawrence, along with his wife, Dr. Lisa Robyn Lawrence, has counseled and treated more than a thousand women with PMS. Dr. Allen Lawrence is presently practicing at The Lawrence Center in Los Angeles, California.

LISA ROBYN LAWRENCE, M.S., PH.D.

Dr. Lisa Robyn Lawrence has worked in the medical field since the age of sixteen. Shortly after meeting Dr. Lawrence it became apparent that PMS was creating a problem in their relationship. It was then that Lisa and Allen Lawrence set out to find the cause and to cure it.

Dr.. Lawrence received a Master's in Women's Nutrition and a Ph.D. in Human Ecology from Pacific Institute for Advanced Studies and her Ph.D. in Human Ecology 1n 1984, Dr. Lisa Robyn Lawrence designed a nutritional program to cure her own PMS. Dr. Together the Lawrence then expanded this program and Dr. Lisa Lawrence been the Director of Nutritional Services for the Reseda Women's Health Center and, subsequently, for the DiversiCare and ActiveCare Medical Group.

Dr. Lisa Lawrence set up and then instituted PMS, prenatal and menopausal nutritional programs within several medical practices. These nutritional programs eventually expanded to also provided nutritional guidance for hyperactive children as well as for people suffering from diabetes, high blood pressure, high cholesterol and general health problems.

Dr. Lisa Robyn Lawrence presently is a consultant and Co-Director and Director of Counseling Services for The Lawrence Center in Los Angeles, California. Dr. Lisa Robyn Lawrence also has a private practice providing a broad range of nutritional counseling including PMS, weight loss, menopause, diabetes mellitus, prenatal, post partum, preeclampsia, hypertension, gastro-esophageal reflux, peptic ulcer and much more.

(This Page Is Purposefully Left Blank For You To Use To Take Notes)

INTRODUCTION

WHAT THE 30-DAYS TO NO MORE PMS PROGRAM CAN DO FOR YOU

Premenstrual Syndrome (PMS) afflicts some 20 to 40 million women each month. Scientific research has established that 40% to 60% of all women between the ages of 19 and 45 already either suffer from PMS or are on their way to developing it. Our 30-Days to No More PMS, PMS Elimination program can help you prevent the many dispiriting symptoms of PMS before they become a significant threat to your physical and emotional health and well-being.

If you are a woman who suffers from PMS and you have been told that PMS is all in your head then our 30-Days to No More PMS program is for you. In it, we will prove conclusively that PMS is real and easily treatable. If you have experienced the Jekyll and Hyde personality changes that occur in the week to two weeks prior to the onset of your menstrual period, this book will be of particular importance to you. Within it we will tell you how to once again take control of your own life.

If you are presently experiencing physically or emotionally debilitating effects from PMS, you will want a fast, easy to use and proven treatment program to reverse, and even eliminate, your symptoms. You will want a program that not only can help you eliminate your PMS symptoms but also teach you how to protect your overall health and well-being.

By using the information provided in our PMS Elimination program, you will be able to rapidly and safely eliminate all of your PMS symptoms.

This information is a must for husbands, mothers, fathers and children of PMS women as well. It is vital information for managers who have PMS women working for them. In fact, for all of those whose lives are negatively affected by PMS, this book will help them understand the problem and show them how to deal with it.

Everything that is presented to you in this 30-Days to No More PMS, Dietary and Nutritional Treatment Program has worked for others. More than a thousand women have used this program to obtain symptom relief. This program works.

When we first developed the 30-Days to No More PMS, Dietary and Nutritional Program, we thought it was our secret system. We believed that its success was dependent specifically on our personal counseling and repeated follow-ups of the women who participated. The diet, we worried, might be so strict and hard to learn that many women would not stay on it.

We soon realized, however, that it was not meant to be a secret system. The program belonged to all women who suffer from PMS. Most of our patients not only did comply with the program, but in fact, most were so delighted with their own success that they soon began teaching it to their daughters, friends and relatives. We also found, over the past 20 years, that once PMS women were able to eliminate their symptoms, they were so relieved that the greatest majority never went back to their old ways of eating. They did not ever want to return to suffering again.

We were also pleased to discover that once PMS symptoms had been eliminated, women could periodically "cheat" on the diet and still remain symptom free. Within our 30-Days to No More PMS program, we will even tell you how to cheat and get away with it.

The original purpose of our program was to educate PMS women, to teach them how to live normal, healthy lives with no PMS symptoms. We were indeed highly successful in doing this. Now we want to teach you so you can eliminate your PMS and make your life more successful than you ever dreamed possible.

Through our research and the development of our counseling program which we are about to
relate to you, we found that PMS is actually a nutritional deficiency syndrome. Once this deficiency is corrected, all of the symptoms that make it up simply disappear.

The underlying concept of this program is that the PMS symptoms you are presently suffering from are an intelligent act of the body designed to tell you that you are eating the wrong foods for your bodily needs. That's right! PMS symptoms are there to tell you that many of the foods you are presently eating may be foods that are not right for your personal needs. As soon as you are able to eat what your body really needs, your PMS symptoms will just go away.

After working with our program for a while, you will be delighted to discover that, in addition to relieving PMS symptoms, this dietary program has many other benefits. For instance, you will find that:

YOU WILL LOOK BETTER AND FEEL MORE VITAL AND ALIVE

Your energy, stamina and ability to function will rise higher than before. Since this program is based on returning to the foods that your body needs the most and eliminating the foods that it does not want, once you are on the right diet for you, you will feel healthier than you have in years. When this happens your energy levels and your ability to function will increase and you will feel wonderful. Our experience has taught us that as a result, your self-confidence will also increase.

Many women have reported an enhanced confidence in their own abilities. Without the monthly PMS symptoms, they have been able to enjoy life more and their sense of self-value and worth increases greatly. Just imagine what a difference this added confidence could make in your life.

When you are no longer under the effects of the symptoms of PMS, you will no longer feel sick, frustrated and out of control during any part of the two weeks prior to your menstrual period. You will no longer have that run-down, bloated, swollen or worn-out feeling. You will no longer have to make excuses and miss out on so many of the joys of life.

As your energy, self-value and self-esteem return, you will feel better about yourself. Life will matter more to you. You will matter more to yourself. Because you feel better, you will want to look better. Once again you will be in charge of your life and life will be worth living.

YOU CAN LOOK FORWARD TO A FULL AND NORMAL LIFE

You can finally start looking ahead to new challenges and more successes in your life. As you feel better about life, you will naturally want more out of life. You will want new experiences. You will want more than ever to succeed in your life. Because you have already won out over your PMS, you may want to take some new risks. When you have experienced success, you will be less afraid of challenges. You will be able to live more in the now-moment. You won't find yourself worrying about either how good or how bad you felt last month or how good or how bad you will feel next month.

By releasing the energy that it took merely to hold your life together while suffering from PMS, you can start feeling great all the time. As you look toward the future, it can now be dedicated to planning and creating new beginnings.

You'll be at your best, ready to tackle life with a new zeal. Having conquered your PMS symptoms and mastered your body, you can now be in charge of your life. This creates a new way of looking at yourself and the life you choose to lead. In the past, the life style you lived and what you ate were the major factors in causing PMS and its limitations. Now, what you choose to eat and how you live your life will remove those limitations and create a new and healthier you. In this new role you will want to grow and flourish, to take new risks and demand more for yourself. You will feel like a winner and you will be ready for just about anything. When you no longer have PMS to pull you down, you can rise to the heights of your personal best. You will have the freedom to realize your highest self.

RELATIONSHIPS CAN IMPROVE BECOME EVEN BETTER

The important, personal relationships with your husband or boyfriend, with your children and with your relatives and friends will become better and more comfortable. When you had your PMS symptoms, you were not always able to be your best self. With PMS gone, you finally can be your best all the time.

When you had PMS, the men in your life may have seen you as unreliable, confusing and unpredictable. During this period of your life you couldn't give the best part of you. But once your PMS symptoms are eliminated, you will be able to give yourself fully to your relationships with your partner and your children. They will see the real, loving, caring, healthy you and your relationships can once again become wholesome and loving.

Making decisions to improve the quality of your life has another side to deal with, your destructive relationships. When PMS sufferers become symptom free, they often realize that many of their relationships have been destructive because of their lack of self-esteem and control over their own emotions. They come to the realization that these relationships either have to be improved or eliminated.

YOUR SEX LIFE CAN BECOME BETTER THAN EVER

While PMS is often associated with increased sexual drive, this does not mean that most PMS women enjoy sex. In fact, you will find that once PMS symptoms are eliminated, sex is considerably better. When you once again can enjoy and appreciate yourself you will find that sex is much more enjoyable. With the dreaded PMS symptoms gone, your stress is reduced and you may find you can allow yourself to once again feel your real emotions, love, caring and self-value. You will now be able, perhaps for the first time in a long while, to let your real self, your sexual self, out to fully enjoy being a woman.

YOU WILL LOOK AND FEEL YOUNGER

In order to eliminate your PMS symptoms, you must learn to eat healthier and better quality foods. When you do this, it can take years off your face and your body. Most women naturally lose weight with little or no effort. Your skin will become enlivened and take on a healthy glow. Your energy levels will rise. Your sense of self-confidence and well-being will dramatically increase. You may look and feel better than you have ever felt before. As the years of suffering fade into the past, the glow of health and your youthful exuberance will return.

YOU WILL BE HEALTHIER

As you eat more healthfully, you will not only feel healthier but actually be healthier. PMS often leads to recurrent illnesses, disabilities and strange symptoms that can rob you of your vitality. With the elimination of PMS, you will feel healthier and more alive than you have in years.

To quickly summarize, PMS is a state of nutritional deficiency. While you are suffering from PMS, you are experiencing the intelligence of your body letting you know that your diet is inadequate for you. By simply changing your diet you can fully and completely eliminate your PMS symptoms forever. Once you are free of PMS, you will be able to be the real you. Your health and well-being will improve. You will look and feel younger. You will have more energy. You will be able to have full and complete charge of your life, you will no longer feel out of control. You will sleep better, eat better, be calmer and have increased sexual vitality. You will be happier and enjoy life more than ever before.

All of this can be yours simply by following this 30-Days to No More PMS Nutritional Program specially designed for you. Are you ready?

Allen Lawrence, MA. M.D., Ph.D.
Lisa Robyn Lawrence, M.S., Ph.D.

Forward

The nature and severity of PMS symptoms vary from woman to woman. Some women may only feel *edgy* or *tired* for a day or two each month. Others may experience such significant and severe discomfort that it interferes with their normal activities anywhere from one day to two or more weeks out of each month.

Until recently, premenstrual complaints were widely considered to be "all in a woman's mind." It is now widely recognized that PMS is real, treatable and specifically related to controllable factors. Our experiences strongly demonstrate to us that diet is the most important factor in both creating and managing PMS.

> *"PMS is a real biologic condition*
> *that is treatable and no woman should have to suffer from it!"*

For many women PMS can rob them of their vitality, energy and well-being. Women lose their jobs because of it. Personal relationships suffer from it. Most women affected by PMS will feel a decreased sense of self-value and self-image. It is not unusual that their families will also suffer severely from the effect of their PMS. Communication between husbands' and wives are often impaired, children are left confused and in extreme cases abused. Many women with PMS will pay the ultimate consequence because of their PMS with divorce, shattered dreams and chaos in their life.

While most women initially have a mild form of PMS, over time PMS is often a progressive condition which can rapidly change and leave women feeling *trapped* in its wake. It is also common that many of these women will have little or no idea of what is happening to them or why it is happening.

If you know that you have PMS you are in a sense lucky for now you can do something about it. In our book, 30-Days to No More PMS, we will look at what PMS is, how it can affect the woman, her family, children and partner. We will look at the symptoms of PMS, and its negative affects and its costs, not just in dollars and cents, but in vitality and quality o life.

HOW WOULD I KNOW IF I HAVE PMS?

PMS can be recognized by the timing of the symptoms and their pattern. Most important is that these symptoms *must occur in the week or two weeks prior to the onset of the menstrual period*. In the following pages we will look at how you can self-diagnose yourself "scientifically." There will be no guess work in it for you will be able to take advantage of our combined 35 years of experience in working with and treating women with PMS.

Before determine whether you have PMS it is important that you learn what PMS is and how to recognize it. The next step is charting your symptoms to establish their pattern and severity. Often professional help may be extremely valuable in evaluating and helping you make a definite diagnosis. Once PMS is diagnosed treatment can be set in motion.

THE FOLLOWING FACTORS CAN MAKE PMS MORE LIKELY:

- Increased Number of Pregnancies
- Age (More common in women 25-35 years of age)
- High Stress Levels or Trauma
- Lack of Exercise
- History of Tubal Ligation
- Use of Birth Control Pills
- Excessive Weight Gain or Loss
- Previous Major Surgeries
- Skipping Meals or Poor Food Choices

IF I HAVE PMS, IS THERE HELP FOR ME?

Today there are many sources for attaining help. Some of these resources can be medical doctors, nutritionists, PMS counselors or health educators. These people can offer medical treatment, alternative medical treatments, counseling and guidance in both managing and eliminating PMS symptoms. Unfortunately, in many cases most PMS sufferers will at best only get quasi good advice and lists of suggestions. For some women this is enough. For most women with moderate to severe PMS this is insufficient and they are unable to eliminate their symptoms without individualized attention and support. In our book, 30-Days to No More PMS, we do not just present suggestions but rather a concrete, tried and proven, program for eliminating symptom and gaining control over your PMS.

30 Days To No More PMS

WHAT IS THE BEST WAY TO TREAT MY PMS?

The single best method of treatment we have found so far is to eat a correct diet. A diet that will correct the nutritional deficiencies and excesses which as you will soon see are causing your PMS symptoms. In most cases, the correction of these nutritional deficiencies completely reverses the PMS symptoms. While some people treat PMS with the female hormone, progesterone and a host of other medications and surgery, we generally suggest against all of these unless it is being used in the most severe cases where both diet and other treatment programs are used together.

Hormonal therapy will help to relive PMS symptoms but it does not reverse the underlying cause of PMS, the nutritional deficiency, and hence while you are left symptom free, you are also left deficient in essential nutrients at the same time. Since the symptoms of PMS are an intelligent communication from your body letting you know that a deficiency exists, covering them up using progesterone, other medications or surgery, simply hides them and leaves you vulnerable to long term health problems.

DO I HAVE TO CHANGE MY DIET RADICALLY?

The answer to this question depends on the individual and the quality of her diet and frequency of her meals or snacks. Since PMS is created by certain deficiencies and excesses in the diet the best way to control PMS is to correct the diet accordingly. In most cases this does require making some dietary changes. We understand that most people do not want to change their life radically. After years of working with women, treating PMS and getting excellent results we can assure you that most all of the women we have worked with are happier and enjoy eating more after their symptoms are gone than they ever did before.

Most of the food choices made while having PMS were driven by cravings that the women did not want to have. Now, with the cravings gone, the former PMS suffer can take control of her life and what she eats.

We also teach you how to cheat periodically so that you can enjoy life to its absolute fullness. So don't worry, you will feel better, healthier and more in control of your life then ever before.

30 Days To No More PMS

Table of Contents

PMS FORMS FOR PERSONAL USE AND TO GIVE TO FRIENDS

TABLES

CHAPTER 1

UNDERSTANDING PREMENSTRUAL SYNDROME (PMS)

Our 30-Days to No More PMS program will show you how to eliminate the symptoms and underlying nutritional deficiencies which cause Premenstrual Syndrome. We will show you how you can get well and stay well simply by learning to choose the best foods to eat for you.

We know that there are numerous medical treatments for PMS. Most of these treatments can, in one way or another, help women relieve some or all of their PMS symptoms. Yet none of these treatments actually solve the problem which causes you to have PMS. You will find as you read further that PMS is a nutritional deficiency syndrome. While other potentially dangerous and costly medical treatments may relieve your symptoms, only the nutritional program presented in our 30-Days to No More PMS program allows you to safely, sanely and rapidly eliminate your PMS symptoms simply by eating healthy, delicious foods. You will find with this program that no medications are necessary and that medical treatment is rarely required.

After all of the years of experience we have had in working with women suffering with PMS, we can certainly understand your discouragement in seeking relief through medical treatment. But we want you to know that it is not necessary for you to endure this any longer. It is now entirely possible to eliminate every single symptom and condition that is related to your PMS quickly and completely. We have worked with more than a thousand women providing them with the information necessary to become symptom free. In case after case, we have seen women, first doubting, then hoping and finally enlivened by the complete disappearance of their PMS symptoms.

We want you to know that if you diligently follow the instructions that we are going to give you, you too can succeed and never again have to suffer the anguish or the health problems associated with PMS.

DR. ALLEN LAWRENCE, A PHYSICIAN'S PERSONAL VIEWPOINT

I can personally relate to the suffering caused by PMS. I became interested in PMS because when Lisa and I met, Lisa suffered severely from PMS. Initially it was through trying to help her overcome her symptoms that I became aware of the extent of the threat of PMS.

Together, Lisa and I learned how to treat her PMS and then how to eliminate it entirely.

As an Obstetrician/Gynecologist I saw many women who suffered from PMS but until my wife and I started working on eliminating her symptoms, I had no idea how devastating PMS could be. Before that I had really believed that the symptoms of PMS were just part of being a woman. Before learning about PMS I believed that all women acted erratically before their menstrual periods. I also believed that PMS was really a form of emotional illness. I now know that this is not true. I want you to know that PMS is real and that, since it is caused by a nutritional deficiency, it is a problem that can be completely eliminated.

DR. LISA LAWRENCE, HER PERSONAL EXPERIENCE WITH PMS

"I was 19 when I first experienced PMS symptoms. After my gynecologist prescribed birth control pills, I began to experience nausea and swelling of my hands and feet. My breasts felt bruised and swollen. I subsequently tried four types of birth control pills but each produced different side effects. The last caused a profound depression. When I went off the pill, I noticed strong cravings for sweets, especially chocolate. I felt like a chocolate vampire. After eating it, I would feel guilty and craved more."

"Throughout the next few years, I would not only become irritable just before my menstrual periods, but I would even provoke arguments. I had headaches, insomnia and fatigue. I was sad and felt very alone. Not trusting my own perceptions, I did not want to make any important decisions at that time of the month. When I told this to my doctor, he told me all he could do for me was prescribe "water pills," for swelling, "sleeping pills" to help me sleep and "nerve pills" to calm me down. All of these medications caused side effects, and the pill to calm me down made me feel so dull and hazy that I could hardly function. I still felt alone and the despair worsened."

"When I spoke to my doctor about these effects, he told me that most of my problems were probably all in my head so I shouldn't really worry. Those words, "all in my head" still ring in my ears."

"Shortly after turning 23, another complication occurred. I detected a lump in my breast. Being told by the surgeon that it had to be surgically removed as soon as possible, I was given a form to sign giving my permission for a possible mastectomy should it be cancerous. I've never been more frightened. Fortunately, the lump was benign, "simply" fibrocystic disease (which I later learned is frequently linked to PMS)."

"During my pregnancy, which occurred a year later, and while breast feeding my son, I was symptom free. But as soon as I weaned him the symptoms of PMS returned, even

2

worse than they had been before. By the time he was two, my marriage was in shambles, my life in confusion and, for two weeks of every month, I couldn't control my life."

"After my divorce I began dating Allen and he and I began to do our research into the cause of my monthly symptoms. Over the next few months, we reviewed all the literature we could find on the subject. We found that PMS most likely is caused by an abnormality in the relationship between estrogen and progesterone. This imbalance, we found, is created by a combination of deficiencies caused by certain foods in our daily diet and by excesses of foods which interfere with the ability of the body to function normally. "

"We formulated a nutritional program which I, myself, followed, and within 30 days of starting the diet, all of my PMS symptoms vanished."

"That was more than 30 years ago and since that time I have had no significant PMS symptoms at all."

MAKING A DECISION TO ELIMINATE YOUR PMS

At this point, we would like to give you some background information which will help you to make the decision to eliminate your symptoms.

It may seem peculiar to you to suggest that you will have to make a conscious decision to free yourself from your PMS symptoms. However, in our many years of clinical experience working with PMS women, we clearly recognize that not all women either want to eliminate their symptoms or are ready to do what is necessary to make it work. The readers of our 30-Days to No More PMS program can be divided into one of three groups:

- Those who will insist on conventional, orthodox medical treatment. That is, the use of medications, drugs and hormones to treat their symptoms. Over the years many women have chosen this course. Generally, we have no difficulty with this choice. Our only reservation is that they are really not treating the cause -- only the symptoms.
- The second group is made up of women who do not want to fully treat their PMS. Even though the women in this group often say that they will try one or more method of treatment, they either do not continue the treatment long enough to get results or they do indeed get results and drop out anyway. These women do not really want to give up their PMS symptoms. They often profess that they do, but their actions generally belie their words.
- The third group is made up of women who want the healthiest and most natural mode of treatment available to eliminate their PMS symptoms. These women are willing

to do whatever is necessary and make it work.

> **There is No Simple One-Step Magic**
>
> **for Curing PMS.**

You may already know which group you belong to. Some women in the first group choose to use conventional medical treatment programs even when they are aware that they are not actually treating the underlying problem and cause. They often do this because they believe that anything outside of orthodox medicine must be "quack" medicine. In a sense, these women have been "brainwashed" and frightened by the medical establishment.

Other women in this group truly believe in the power of medicine. For them, nothing can cure their problems unless it comes in the form of a pill or possibly a surgical procedure. Still, other women don't want to work at trying to eliminate their PMS. The idea of having to think, plan and be responsible for their actions is quite disturbing. For these women it is much simpler to just do what their doctors tell them to do rather than to think for themselves. However, there is no drug or chemical product which will cure Premenstrual Syndrome.

Those doctors--and patients--who believe that PMS can be eliminated by a pill or a potion simply are fooling themselves. The medical prescriptive methods simply cover up the symptoms of PMS. They do not cure them. They are expensive. They can have dangerous side effects. They require you to have ongoing medical care. And they keep you from truly being in control of your own life and destiny. You might think that we are being hard on the medical profession, but we are not, we are just being honest.

For fear of being ridiculed by their friends, family or their doctors, some women won't even try alternative methods. They may be afraid that if they do not follow exactly what their doctor tells them, the doctor will be angry at them, and possibly even reject them. They may feel that their doctor knows what is best for them and so they blindly follow his plan for them. They may even feel that since they are paying for his advice, they owe it to him regardless of what may actually be in their own best interests.

We truly feel sorry for these women as they work hard at making sure that no one gets hurt but themselves. They often do not look closely at the record of the medical profession when it comes to cures. They don't notice that few people ever get cured by medical treatment of chronic illnesses and problems like PMS. Most simply get treated...for the rest of their lives.

One last comment about this group. Some get pulled into it because they believe that they can't afford alternative methods. They get their doctor's visits and their medications paid for through their insurance plans. And they believe that they are unable to afford counseling and care outside of the medical system.

We used to run into this conflict often. Women would call and ask questions about treating their PMS but they belonged to an HMO or managed care program that would not provide PMS counseling services. Often, rather than paying to learn how to eat the right foods to eliminate their PMS, they would opt to make use of their health plan and take what they were given. They often did this even after we told them that the cost of counseling would be more than made up for by their savings in buying more healthful and nutritious foods.

The readers of our 30-Days to No More PMS program will not have to worry about the cost of medical care, nor who they make happy other than themselves. Within this book, we will give you virtually all the information you will need to eliminate all of your PMS symptoms and all you will have to do is eat your way back to good health and freedom from PMS.

To point out the hazards women face when they choose traditional medicine to treat their PMS, we would like to give you some examples of the kinds of medical treatments commonly prescribed. See for yourself whether they make sense to you.

Many physicians prescribe medications simply to eliminate the symptoms of PMS without ever eliminating the reason for PMS. Diuretics or water pills are commonly prescribed. Since swelling of the hands and feet, upper and lower extremities, face and breasts are common symptoms with PMS, water pills are used to expel water from the system. While they often do work for many women, they don't work for every woman. They are extremely harsh on the body, forcing water from the tissues and blood to be excreted by the kidneys.

Many women can become deficient in a very important mineral called potassium. Potassium deficiency can cause fatigue, weakness, dizziness, an irregular heart rate and occasionally collapse. It may require taking more pills to replace the lost potassium or eating foods high in potassium which if they are the wrong foods can intensify their PMS symptoms.

Frequently tranquilizers, mood elevators and antidepressants are used to control the mood of the PMS woman. Sleeping pills are often prescribed to help PMS women get to sleep and occasionally amphetamines are prescribed to wake them up.

Hormones, particularly estrogen, which can alter the normal cyclic function of the body, may be prescribed even though irregular bleeding is a common side effect.

Some women are placed on birth control pills which in fact may worsen their symptoms. Commonly the hormone progesterone is prescribed in the form of rectal or vaginal suppositories. While it often works to eliminate PMS symptoms, it is generally quite messy, irritating, inconvenient and costly.

We will discuss many of these methods of treatment in a later chapter but we thought it would be of value to have an overview of the medical treatments even before we get into the dietary method of treating PMS.

The women of the second group discussed above--those who are either unwilling or not ready to treat their PMS--are another interesting group. While PMS often causes these women significant problems, they may not be able to avail themselves of treatment. There are a number of important reasons for this. Many of these reasons overlap the first group to some degree.

Many women don't believe that they can get relief from their symptoms so they feel that trying would only be painful and that they will probably fail anyway. They are either afraid to fail or they are afraid to succeed.

Some women need their PMS symptoms. These women get a certain kind of secondary gain from having PMS. It may be that it gives them a reason to rationalize their failures. If they can't eliminate their PMS symptoms, they will never have to find out whether their PMS is the reason they fail at everything or whether underneath they are really a failure.

In some women, their PMS symptoms help them to control husbands, partners, children, family, employers or employees. Eliminating their PMS symptoms might eliminate their advantage.

While it may seem almost preposterous that logic like this could exist, this group of women clearly demonstrates that it does in fact exist. At the risk of seeming judgmental, we believe that it is important to point this out. The women of this group deserve a clear message that holding on to their PMS symptoms is foolish. It is as foolish as using dangerous methods of treatment to protect your doctor or to prevent ridicule. Many women each year go untreated or are inadequately treated for the above reasons.

The third group, and it is likely that you belong to it since you have purchased our 30-Days to No More PMS program, is the healthiest of all. The women of this group are willing to do whatever is necessary to rid themselves of their PMS symptoms.

Since the women of this group are usually quite intelligent and discerning, it is likely that they would want to know what our nutritional method is, how it works and why they should use it.

Please be patient, for in the next chapters we will give you all of the information you will need to help you get the results you desire. We will also give you all the information you need to make it work--painlessly, effortlessly, and we might add, deliciously.

However, before we start this part of the discussion, we believe that we must first tell you what PMS is, how you recognize it, who gets it and how you get it. This, therefore, must be our next task.

In the course of this discussion we will give you some case histories of women, just like yourself, who suffered PMS and who, through the help of our dietary program, are now symptom free.

SYMPTOMS OF PMS

Premenstrual Syndrome (PMS) can best be understood as a group of symptoms that occur in affected women in the second half of the menstrual cycle. These symptoms can last as long as two weeks or as briefly as one day. They always occur prior to the onset of menstruation and disappear either immediately upon the onset of menstrual bleeding or shortly thereafter.

PMS can occur in any woman between the ages of 19 and 45 years old. The youngest person we know of suffering from PMS was a 14-year-old and the oldest was 50 years of age. Estimates suggest that there could be as many as 20-40 million women in America who suffer from PMS. We believe that some 30% to 40% of these women have symptoms that significantly interfere with their ability to function normally, take care of themselves or their families or which interfere with their performance on the job.

In younger women, PMS symptoms tend to be quite mild, but with time the symptoms can become considerably more severe. By the time most PMS women reach the age of 25 to 35, their symptoms will have reached their greatest intensity.

There are four groups of symptoms which are seen most commonly: the PMS - A or *Anxiety Group*, the PMS - H or *Hydrous or Water Group*, the PMS - C or *Cravings Group* and finally, the PMS - D or *Depression Group*. (See Table 1.)

THE PMS - A, ANXIETY GROUP

The PMS - A, *Anxiety Group*, includes a number of primary symptoms which torment women with anxiety, mood swings, irritability and nervous tension. This is the most common group of symptoms associated with PMS. Nearly 80% of PMS women have symptoms attributed to PMS A Group to some degree. These symptoms often start as early as two

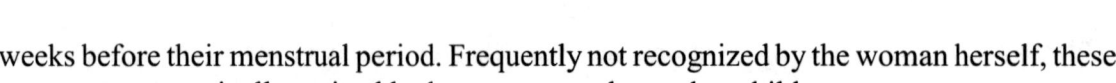

weeks before their menstrual period. Frequently not recognized by the woman herself, these symptoms are typically noticed by her partner and even her children.

Most Common PMS Symptoms

PMS-A
Anxiety Group

Anxiety
Mood Swings
Irritability
Nervous Tension

PMS-H
Hydrous (Water) Group

Weight Gain
Swelling of Extremeties
Breast Tenderness
Abdominal Bloating

PMS-C
Craving Group

Headaches
Craving for Sweets
Increased Appetite
Heart Pounding
Fatigue
Dizzyness or Fainting

PMS-D
Depression Group

Depression
Forgetfulness
Crying
Confusion
Insomina

Table 1

As one patient's husband once told us, "We always know that when Margaret starts into her 'meanie week,' she is due for her menstrual period."

These symptoms are related to elevated levels of the female hormone, estrogen. This elevation, as we will soon find out, is created by a relatively high dietary intake of foods high in sugar, simple carbohydrates and calcium. We will discuss this relationship in much greater detail in the chapter on the nutritional basis for PMS.

These symptoms are often stimulated and made worse by stress of any kind.

PMS - H OR HYDROUS, WATER GROUP

More than 60% of all PMS women have PMS, suffer from PMS - H or *Hydrous, Water Group*. The primary symptoms of this group are weight gain, swelling of the extremities, breast tenderness and abdominal bloating. These symptoms and physical changes commonly undermine the self-image of the PMS-H women. The swelling is usually seen as getting "fatter" and this weakens her self-value. When the PMS woman who is already very emotionally distressed sees herself swelling and gaining weight, she is often driven to starve herself. This ultimately leads to overwhelming hunger and binging, and then to trying to control weight gain through either purging or to the chronic use of laxatives.

THE PMS - C, CRAVINGS GROUP

The PMS - C, *Cravings Group* is the next largest, occurring in 40% of all women with PMS. The primary symptoms in this group are craving for sweets, increased appetite, headaches, pounding heart, fatigue and dizziness or fainting. It is referred to as the cravings group because most of the symptoms relate to either increased appetite or cravings for certain foods during the week to two weeks prior to the onset of menstruation. The most prominent craving is for chocolate but for many PMS women the cravings can be for anything that is sweet. Generally the cravings come in times of increased stress, but ultimately can come at anytime during the week or two before the onset of the next menstrual period.

When the PMS woman feels tense or stressed, and this is during a good portion of the PMS period, she may feel that the only thing that relieves her tension is eating. Sweets seem to do the job best but any food will usually do if sweets are unavailable. Once she is through indulging herself, she usually feels fatigued, somewhat down, her heart may pound, she may get the shakes and very often she gets a severe, throbbing headache. On occasion, she may feel dizzy. She may feel faint or even faint. In any case, she usually feels guilty for indulging and frustrated with the cravings.

These symptoms are also related to elevated estrogen and excess insulin release caused by the increased sugar she has consumed. The elevated estrogen levels create changes in the chemistry of the brain and these changes create the cravings for sugar. This combination of events causes major problems for this group and leads to great frustration.

THE PMS - D, DEPRESSION GROUP

The PMS - D, *Depression Group* occurs only in about 20% of all women who suffer from PMS. It most commonly occurs in association with the anxiety group. This group includes a number of highly disabling symptoms such as depression, withdrawal, forgetfulness, frequent crying, confusion and insomnia.

This group can be of special concern, for it is common for women with this group of symptoms to have suicidal thoughts and actually become a danger to themselves. Occasionally they may even attempt suicide. And, tragically, sometimes they succeed.

This group differs from the other three groups in that it may be due to low levels of estrogen rather than elevated levels of estrogen as is true in the other groups. It is worsened by giving progesterone and may best be helped in the short run, either by giving oral or injectable estrogen, or using antidepressants, particularly the serotonin reuptake inhibitors which we will talk about in a later section.

FREQUENT SYMPTOMS	
Dr. Katherina Dalton Lists The Following Symptoms As Common:	
Psychological:	Lethargy, feeling suicidal, moodiness, personality changes, assault, child abuse, self injury, alcoholic addictions, anxiety, panic.
Neurological:	Migraine, epilepsy, vertigo or dizziness.
Dermatological:	Acne, boils, herpes, urticaria (hives).
Respiratory:	Asthma, rhinitis (runny nose).
Orthopedic:	Backache, joint pains, edema (swelling).
Ophthalmologic:	Sties, conjunctivitis (pink eye), glaucoma, uveitis (infection of the uvea of the eye.)
Otorhinolaryngology:	Sinusitis, sore throat, hoarseness.
Urologic:	Cystitis (bladder infections), urethritis (urethral infection).
Gastro-Intestinal:	Abdominal pains, compulsive eating, diarrhea and constipation.
Mammology:	Breast engorgement and swelling.

Table 2

While we have divided up the symptoms listed into groups, we must make it clear that any one individual may have a potpourri of symptoms. She does not necessarily have all of the symptoms of any group and she may have a varying degree of symptoms from one or all four groups.

10

To date more than 150 different symptoms have been recognized and attributed to PMS. PMS symptoms are found to involve just about every organ and organ system of the body. Symptoms of PMS range from mild mood changes all the way to serious suicidal behavior; from acne to alcoholism.

Characteristic of the change in eating habits frequently seen in PMS victims are uncontrollable food binges and an inability to stop eating, especially chocolate or other sweets. This overeating, along with fluid retention, leads to swelling and weight gain.
There is a very definite alteration of the PMS woman's tolerance for alcohol, predominately just before her menstrual periods start. Alcohol acts like sugar. Feeling poorly, the PMS woman may be drawn to use alcohol in order to raise her brain and blood sugar but the body burns it up so rapidly that she can never quite get enough.

MORE DIFFICULT TO RECOGNIZE SYMPTOMS:
This Is a Group of Symptoms Not Often Recognized as Due to PMS

- Uncontrollable food binging
- Inability to stop eating chocolate or sweets
- Altered tolerance to alcohol just before menstruation, alcoholism
- Increased or decreased libido and sexuality, nymphomania
- Difficulty sleeping, insomnia
- Taking naps or not able to get out of bed
- Decreased feeling of well-being
- Distractable and difficulty coping with life
- Need for affection, to give and receive it
- Orderliness, even compulsiveness
- Bursts of energy and activity
- Aggression, impulse to harm to others
- Lowered performance and self-esteem
- Feelings of unworthiness and diminished self-value
- Difficulty communicating with others

- Impaired judgement
- Difficulty in concentration
- Inability to cope with work
- Easily excitable even high strung or emotional
- Feelings of loss of control
- Avoidance of social interaction
- Restlessness
- Change in eating habits
- Hopelessness and despair
- Surges of fear and even phobias
- Anxiety or panic attacks, agoraphobia
- Fear of death, fantasies of death or suicide
- Loneliness or wanting to be alone and avoid others
- Need for frequent or even constant reassurance

Table 3

Initially, she may need one drink to feel good, however within a short while she may need several drinks to maintain even a slight feeling of well-being. Many PMS women inadvertently become alcoholics because of this mechanism.

Women with PMS often have difficulty sleeping. This difficulty seems exaggerated because throughout the day and into the night their minds seem to be going virtually nonstop. They also often feel anxious or depressed, sometimes both at the same time.

PMS women often experience sudden bursts of energy and activity and extreme excitement. They may experience periods of restlessness or profound fatigue during the day. They may need to take naps on and off to compensate for this fatigue. When they finally are able to fall asleep, they may have highly emotional dreams which wake them, further disturbing their sleep. Often, once in bed and asleep they have extreme difficulty waking up in the morning.

When a PMS woman is functionally impaired, her impairment tended to be greatest in her own home, but is quickly followed by impairment in social, school, and occupational situations. Among working women, more than 50% of PMS women reported being at least somewhat lowered occupational functioning. Of women who at one point or another had missed work because of their symptoms, between 1 and 7 days were missed within the past year of their employment. Almost three-fourths of the women studied had never sought treatment, and the severity of their symptom was a very important factor as to whether or not they finally sought any form of treatment, medical or alternative.

In Chapter 2 we will introduce you to the hormonal changes that are responsible for PMS. The major defect we will demonstrate is an imbalance between the female hormones' estrogen and progesterone. These are the female sex hormones. If the female sex hormones are interfered with, then sexual feelings and sexual behavior might also be affected. It is common for PMS women to report an alteration in their ability to be affectionate, in increased or decreased sexuality and sexual activity. In teenage girls, increased or hypersexuality, occasionally bordering on nymphomania, appears to be a quite distressing symptom of PMS. With this increase sexual acting out the risk of unwanted pregnancy or acquiring a sexually transmitted disease, with pelvic infection and later sterility is always a potential problem related to uncontrolled PMS.

PMS often predispose women to strong surges of fear, aggression, an impulse to harm others, lowered performance and low self-esteem. The PMS woman may have difficulty communicating with others. She may be prone to feelings of loneliness or wanting to be alone. She may avoid interaction with other people and social situations.

The PMS woman may experience episodes of impaired judgement, difficulty concentrating and an inability to cope with work. She is also prone to increased feelings of worthlessness, hopelessness and despair. She may suffer feelings of loss of control. As we have described above, many personality changes are noted including increased combativeness, incidence of assaulting others, increased risk of becoming a child, husband or parental abuser and have a higher risk of self injury or mutilation. These personality changes may lead to severe conflict for the PMS woman and significantly increase the likelihood of anxiety reactions and even panic attacks. Emotions are not just present, but exaggerated to their extremes. Up is really up and down is really down with PMS.

Fear of death, fantasies of death or suicide and phobic behavior may occur. They may happen as a result of some of the other personality changes or as a reaction to certain physical symptoms.

Along with the many emotional and physical symptoms discussed above, a number of illnesses and medical conditions seem to be cyclically associated with PMS. These conditions are not caused by PMS but rather are triggered either by the emotional reactions or the biochemical changes that undermines her immune system. These conditions are particularly responsive to increased stress. They affect virtually every organ system in the body.

Some of the most commonly seen medical conditions are: allergy, acne, boils, herpes (when infection already exists), hives, runny nose, asthma, sties, conjunctivitis and other eye infections, glaucoma, sinus infections, sore throat, hoarseness, laryngitis, abdominal pains, infections of the bladder and urethra, backache, joint pains, tension headaches, migraine headaches and even epileptic seizures.

It should certainly be clear by now why PMS women are subject to such profound negative feelings -- why they have a decreased sense of well-being and experience such difficulty coping with life. PMS is not just a nuisance or an annoying situation that some women must face. It can be a severe debilitating and disruptive condition that must be eliminated.

Not all women experience the severity of symptoms we have described above. However, many women who read our *30-Days to No More PMS* program may find that the symptoms they experience today will worsen in the next few years. It has also been our experience that many PMS women are unable to recognize the degree of their own disability.

Summary of Factors Involved In PMS	
Factor	**Summary**
Diet	Poor diet is the most important factor in worsening the symptoms and possibly the course of PMS.
Age	PMS tends to worsen with advancing age. Women in the thirties tend to be most commonly to have symptoms.
	Is PMS inherited? It appears to follow family lines.
Marital Status	Married women complain more of PMS symptoms than do single women. PMS is a major cause of divorce and marital stress.
Stress	PMS causes stress and is also made worse by stress and stressful situations.
Pregnancy	PMS tend to increase with the number of pregnancies and births.
Activity/Physical Exercise	Lack of physical activity worsens PMS.
Oral Contraceptives	Birth control pills will tend to worsen the symptoms of PMS in some women and decrease PMS symptoms in other women.
Post Tubal Ligation	Post Tubal Ligation Syndrome consists of: pelvic pain, irregular bleeding, PMS.
Surgery	Any surgery may trigger PMS symptoms.
Weight Gain/Loss	Weight changes of 20-30 lbs. in relatively short periods of time (excluding pregnancy) may trigger PMS.
Lifestyle	Your lifestyle, use of alcohol, degree of rest, stress, how you relate to your family.
Work	The type of job you do, how long and how hard you work.
Trauma	Any trauma may trigger PMS symptoms.

Table 4

PREMENSTRUAL DYSPHORIC DISORDER - PMDD

Premenstrual Dysphoric Disorder or PMDD, is a medical condition that affects millions of women. Premenstrual PMDD however, is viewed as an extreme form of PMS and has been classified as a form of mental illness. The definition of PMDD requires that the woman has at least five out of 10 symptoms and one core symptom must be present, including depressed mood, anxiety, tension and emotional liability. Depression is the most common symptom attributed to this mood disorder, however, abnormal levels of anxiety, anger, sadness, grief, rage or elation are also often considered to be involved with a PMS mood disorder that would be considered to be a PMDD problem. PMDD is usually also based on the timing of its symptoms, a personal estimation of severity of these symptoms (generally the exact same list of symptoms as you will find in Tables 1, 2 and 3), and some form of monitoring of the symptoms to verify the timing and severity of the symptoms. Like PMS, PMDD must occur in the week to two weeks period prior to the onset of menstruation and it must disappear a few days thereafter. However, PMDD symptoms go far beyond what are considered manageable and beyond normal premenstrual symptoms. PMDD is characterized as *severe* monthly mood swings and physical symptoms that interfere with everyday life, especially a woman's relationships with her family and friends. Also like PMS the symptoms and their severity may vary from month to month.

FACTORS PREDISPOSING TO THE CREATION OF PMS

There are a number of factors which appear to increase a woman's risk of getting PMS. The first and possibly most important is diet. These factors do not affect all women equally. Any one factor may play a more important role, in the establishment of PMS, for one woman than it does in another. (See Table 4, above.)

Each of these factors impacts women differently. They cannot be compared uniformly in judging their effects upon the creation of PMS or upon its severity. However, these factors do play a significant role and should be discussed.

Diet

While all of the factors we will discuss play important roles in the creation of PMS, none is more important than diet. We will look carefully at the foods we eat, how they affect us and what we can do about this.

We have already acknowledged that diet is possibly the most important factor involved in the creation of PMS, and we will discuss this in much greater depth in the next chapter. What we will describe is no secret by this time. A diet rich in highly nutritious foods, also vitamins and minerals which oppose PMS and lead to the complete elimination of all symptoms and other problems associated with PMS. On the other hand, a diet which is deficient in essential nutrients, or in "good foods" or contains a lot of "offender foods," can provoke or generate PMS. This type of diet will worsen not only the symptoms of PMS, but often its entire course.

In order to explain the reasoning behind the use of a nutritional approach, it is necessary for us to present a great deal of information about the foods you eat, how they cause PMS and the foods you can eat that will eliminate it. We believe that this information will help the reader of our 30-Days to No More PMS to quickly eliminate their PMS symptoms.

Age

Age seems to play an important role in PMS. PMS unquestionably tends to worsen with advancing age. While PMS often begins in the early twenties, it may not become severe enough to be registered as a problem until the woman reaches her thirties. The most common time for PMS women to seek help is between the ages of twenty-five and thirty-five. Once again, these facts are not in conflict with a nutritional cause. As the PMS woman gets older, if she doesn't clear up her diet, the degree of her nutritional deficiencies will gradually worsen and so will her PMS symptoms.

Family History

Although it is often seen where no family history can be established, PMS appears to run in families, especially on the maternal side. This indicates the possibility that the underlying cause of PMS may have a genetic basis. That is, some women may have a greater predisposition and likelihood of developing PMS because of a gene passed from mother to daughter. While heredity appears to be a factor, specific symptoms may differ significantly between her, her sisters, her mother or her daughters. It would appear that some women have a more fragile response to small deficiencies of particular nutrients while others do not. This genetic factor would tend to stimulate the creation of PMS, however, it is likely that it is the deficiency-excess diet which we will discuss in greater detail, that acts as the final trigger to actually cause the PMS symptoms.

Also mothers' teach their daughters' how and what to eat so there may be an increased tendency toward nutritional deficiency if her mother is a PMS sufferer, and she may teach her daughters to have PMS. This is another reason sisters might also have PMS. Finally, mothers' can teach daughters to be emotional and have many PMS-like symptoms even though the daughter actually may not actually have full-blown PMS. This can be a learned behavior which is not caused by real PMS.

Marital Status

Living with a spouse or roommate appears to play a role in PMS. These women seem to complain more often of PMS symptoms than do single women who live alone. Most statistics in early studies suggested that married women were more prone to PMS. However, recent studies do not show this same result. It has been our experience that the woman who suffers from PMS does not always recognize that she has PMS. Often our most severe PMS patients were brought in by their husbands or other family members. Many of these women refused to admit that *they* had a problem.

It is our belief that women who have PMS are not always aware of the scope and importance of their symptoms. This may account for the reason why in the early studies of PMS, women were less likely to identify with it. Unless they were being told by their husbands that they had a problem, they were not always able to recognize it easily. Hence single women living alone may have had just as high an incidence but no one to reflect off of.

Another factor that has been suggested is that married women have different diets and stress levels than single women. Single women also may have fewer children, etc. As we have seen no appreciable difference in recent years, we do not take much interest in all these arguments. A fact that does seem important to mention is that PMS appears to be a major cause of divorce and marital stress. However, to date, no study has been done to correlate successful treatment of PMS and preservation of marriages.

Stress

PMS affects both women and their families. It is a major cause of marital breakup and divorce. PMS causes stress in relationship to relationship, children, job, self-image, self-worth and self-value. PMS will ultimately not only cause stress, but it can also worsen already existing stress. Stress causes muscle and body tension and long-standing tension then creates fatigue, distraction, difficulty sleeping and getting to sleep (insomnia), but also feelings of illness, muscle and stomach aches and pains, headaches, lowering of your ability to fight and resist illness and to resist the onset and worsening of many chronic diseases. These symptoms when added to the existing PMS symptoms can often cause even the strongest woman to lose hope and fear failure.

Once stress exists the tension it creates is often very difficult to release, however release of tension is ultimately extremely important if the PMS woman is to get lasting relief. If, on the other hand, stress cannot be eliminated, stress is also unlikely to be eliminated. And even if the actual stressor itself is eliminated this is no guarantee that already existing chronic tension can be easily dissipated. When the PMS woman is unaware that she is chronically stressed this can ultimately lead her to mistakenly believe that the therapeutic program, whatever it is, is less effective than it actually may be. Hence, the woman may give up treating her PMS and not return to obtain the much needed help she really should have. Often therapeutic programs are of much lower value because of the PMS women is not entirely in control of her body, her muscles or her nervous system. If she could get past the many stresses in her life, her PMS might respond a lot better and a lot faster.

When the stressed PMS woman is only treated with prescription medication, for example diuretics, tranquilizers, mood elevators, anti-depressants, anti-inflammatory agents or birth control pills, it may in most circumstances make her PMS worse or cause menstrual irregularities. This is because these treatments often act as additional stressors, but more importantly, because the real underlying causes of her PMS, her diet, and the stresses that undermine her, are not directly being treated. On the other hand, if she is placed on a good healthy diet of whole foods, with elimination of PMS trigger foods and a program of exercise, and her stresses are addressed, her PMS is very likely to also improve.

Stress is best relieved by finding the underlying faulty beliefs and fears that cause it. This is often best done in a form of individual or family therapy with a therapist how actually knows what they are doing. Stress can also be reduced and tension temporarily eliminated or decreased under the care of a competent body worker, massage therapist, biofeedback therapist who have the skill, the time, and the interest. Counseling, education and instruction in dietary techniques and exercise will also help. Unfortunately, most of this is not covered by insurance and most women do not have the financial wherewithal to get the results they really need. Yet, stress reduction programs are available in workshops, group programs, books and tape. In many cases these can help a lot.

Stress is one of the most powerful forces in creating or worsening PMS. The stress mechanism itself requires many of the exact same vitamins and minerals that are needed to manage the hormonal and metabolic actions that when out of balance lead to PMS. The B vitamins are very important in this process. Magnesium is so important that it is often called the anti-stress mineral.

Pregnancy

The likelihood of getting PMS seems to increase greatly with the number of pregnancies and births the PMS woman has had. The tendency appears to increase as the number of pregnancies (including miscarriages, abortions, and full term births) increase. This is not at all inconsistent with the nutritional deficiency theorem. With each pregnancy the need for B vitamins and magnesium, as well as most other essential vitamins and minerals, increases because of the greater needs of the mother's body and of the fetus itself. The same is true of lactation -- breast feeding also increases the mother's need for these substances.

If the woman's diet is deficient before pregnancy or becomes deficient during pregnancy it is likely that the woman will be deficient after her pregnancy is completed. In fact she may even be more depleted after pregnancy than she was before. Therefore, if she had a tendency toward PMS before her pregnancy, it is likely that her symptoms will worsen later. Indeed this is exactly what we see. Women with mild PMS symptoms before pregnancy often experience more severe symptoms afterward.

In our practice, however, we worked with PMS women, helping them to become symptom free before they become pregnant. Women who were pregnant when they came to us, and who had suffered from PMS prior to getting pregnant, were treated by placing them on our nutritional program and supplements. In this group of more than a hundred such women, none has had PMS symptoms afterward. None of them has experienced pre-eclampsia (toxemia) of pregnancy nor any excessive weight gain, edema, post-partum depression or even post-partum blues.

Activity/Physical Exercise

This is an especially important factor. In some situations, lack of physical activity can worsen PMS symptoms. Increased physical activity, especially outdoor activity, tends to improve PMS symptoms. There are a number of reasons why this is so. The most important one is that during exercise the body releases *endorphins*. A group of natural morphine-like chemicals, endorphins increase our sense of well-being. These endorphins reduce sensations of pain, fatigue and depression. They are the body's natural way of dealing with these symptoms.

Another reason exercise makes one feel better is that it releases stress and increases relaxation. After physical exercise we naturally relax our entire body and even the stresses we felt prior to exercising are relieved. Finally, the diet is often subtly or dramatically changed due to the increased needs of the body caused by exercising. In addition, the woman who feels healthier often eats more healthfully. Mental relaxation exercises can also have a very similar effect upon our body.

Oral Contraceptives

Birth control pills as they are frequently known, all contain synthetic progesterone, called *progestogens* and as you will soon see progestogens tend to worsen the symptoms of PMS. Birth control pills, often referred to as BCP's, also contain very potent synthetic estrogens. These can further raise estrogen levels and worsen PMS symptoms. The BCP's work by creating a state of pseudo-pregnancy (false pregnancy) and, because of this, many metabolic changes occur which may potentiate PMS. It is common to see women having almost continuous, daily, PMS symptoms while taking certain BCP's.

We are not against the use of BCP's for contraception in a woman who also suffers from PMS, but rather suggest careful observation and, of course, an excellent anti-PMS diet while on them. If a woman doesn't want to become pregnant at any given time or wishes to postpone pregnancy until she is ready, using BCP's may be best overall for her. This decision should always be balanced by her response to the medication and how it affects her PMS.

Post Tubal Ligation

Hysterectomy or tubal ligation may be a predisposing factor to hormonal problems including PMS. Many women who have tubal ligations done, especially by laparoscopy, may later develop post-tubal ligation syndrome. The syndrome consists of a triad of symptoms and complaints including: pelvic pain, irregular bleeding and PMS. The exact nature of post-tubal ligation syndrome is not known but experts believe that interruption of the blood from the ovary directly to the uterus (and vice versa) may somehow be at fault. Any women who has PMS should be concerned and start an anti-PMS diet prior to having a tubal ligation. This would be an important step to take whether the procedure is performed immediately after delivery, in the post-partum period or unrelated to pregnancy.

Surgery

While having had a tubal ligation or hysterectomy appears to increase the risk of triggering PMS, any surgery can in fact, trigger PMS symptoms. Surgery often occurs at the end of an associated illness. Over the period of the illness, changes in dietary habits may occur. These changes might include not eating well, eating more easily digested foods (usually processed foods or simple carbohydrates) or drinking fluids only. It is the intake of processed foods, simple carbohydrates and other minimally nutritious foods which predispose a woman to PMS.

While undergoing surgery and in the post operative phase, intravenous glucose and other fluids present a problem. Not only do they contain no anti-PMS substances, they are essentially pure sugar or entirely devoid of nutrients. Surgery itself is clearly a stressor and almost always triggers the stress mechanism. This certainly increases the likelihood of problems with PMS later.

In the recovery phase, the diet may be extremely limited. The patient is still stressed as the body heals. The fluid shifts that occurred during the illness and surgery must equalize out and resolve themselves. And this places an added strain on the body. Often there is a substantial loss of appetite and subsequent weight loss.

Friends and relatives bring chocolates, candy and fast foods. In the process of recovering from her ordeal, the convalescent may feel justified in eating these less nutritious foods. The internal trauma created by the illness and surgery may have caused enormous metabolic changes. As the recovery progresses, these metabolic changes may potentiate or lead to an increase of PMS symptoms.

Occasionally, a post-surgical depression may occur. This depression may be very similar in nature to post-partum depression. Post-partum depression is now recognized as related to PMS. However, few experts would be willing at this point to admit that many women who suffer post-surgical depression may well be undergoing the same type of phenomena: the effects of nutritional deficiencies related to illness and surgery.

Weight Gain or Loss Is Often Associated with PMS

Weight changes of 20-30 pounds in relatively short periods of time (excluding pregnancy) may trigger PMS. Often dieting is associated with starvation or severe food deprivation. This may accentuate existing deficiencies of B vitamins and magnesium. Excessive weight gain is often associated with an increased intake of fats and simple carbohydrates. This means that the diet is either relatively or absolutely deficient in nutrients which can protect against PMS.

Life Style

The way people live their life is often extremely important. How we live our life often affects our physical and biologic processes. Women who do not eat regularly, who skip meals, eat junk foods or high fat diets, diet frequently to lose weight, use alcohol more than occasionally, eat sweets (especially chocolate), are under stress or who do not get adequate sleep or rest are at greater risk for having PMS. They also will tend to have more severe symptoms. Just as increased physical activity decreases PMS symptoms, lack of physical activity can increase PMS symptoms.

Work

The type of job the PMS woman has, whether in the home, factory, office or boardroom, can affect her level of stress, her diet and her ability to exercise. Along with her job comes her need to be a wife and mother, a daughter and friend. When she is able to balance all of these roles, she may well be able to control her PMS. However, when she is unable to balance all of these roles, it is likely that she is neither able to control her life nor her PMS. Besides the influence of the job on PMS, there is also an effect of PMS on the job. Several studies have suggested that there could be hundreds of thousands, or even millions, of dollars lost by industry each year because of employees suffering from PMS. This occurs as a result of lost time, injuries, increased medical costs, absenteeism, loss of productivity and diminished performance. Once again, there are no studies to indicate what effect proper treatment of PMS might have on business and industry.

Trauma

Any major trauma may trigger PMS symptoms. Surgeries which we discussed above are traumatic to the body. Significant stress is often generated by traumas. At times significant dietary changes may be associated with significant trauma. The greater the trauma, the greater the potential for an increase of PMS. Severe trauma may include hospitalization, food deprivation and/or an increase in the consumption of simple carbohydrates and processed foods. Life threatening traumas may distort the metabolic system for months or years after the trauma.

Painful Menstruation

Painful menstruation, also called dysmenorrhea, is not a symptom of PMS. We have added this section here to note that this condition is often confused with PMS, but it is not directly related to

PMS. As you will see in a later section that pain which occurs just before or during the menstrual cycle may be caused by endometriosis. While endometriosis may be related to PMS, the normal pains associated with menstruation are not at all related to PMS. Often women think that this is one of the main symptoms of PMS, but once again it is not. Women who have PMS may also experience menstrual cramping and suffer from dysmenorrhea. However, while many PMS sufferers have experienced noticeable relief from their menstrual discomfort when treated with the nutritional-dietary approach for PMS, dysmenorrhea sufferers generally does not respond to PMS treatment.

CASE HISTORY #1

When they first came to us seeking help, Martha and Joe N. were both in their early thirties. Joe had literally forced Martha to seek medical attention for her PMS. He told us that in the week and a half before her menstrual period Martha was prone to fits of depression. He stated that she was also so forgetful that on several occasions she had inadvertently set the house on fire by putting down burning cigarettes on tables and close to drapes and other flammable materials. She would, at times, forget to feed their children and clean their house.

She would often have fits of crying and rage and on several occasions she had experienced severe panic attacks. Most disconcerting of all, she would forget that these episodes even happened shortly after they were over.

Martha proved to be eager to learn as much as she could about PMS. She realized that her relationship was in desperate trouble because of her PMS, when she didn't know what to do she felt helpless but as soon as we told her that her PMS was 100% treatable and could be eliminated she was relieved and joined into helping herself.

Martha was very lucky for her husband Joe was extremely supportive. Together they learned what needed to be done and put it into action. Within 2 months Martha was entirely symptom free. The process of working together strengthened their relationship. The last time we saw Martha and Joe, Joe thanked us by saying, "I can't thank you both enough, I finally have my real Martha back again."

CASE HISTORY #2

Sue R. had an excellent job as Director of Sales for a major hotel chain. She suffered from severe PMS but for a number of years was able to control her symptoms. She would selectively arrange her schedule so that it was relatively light, so that she wouldn't have to go out of town or have major projects during her PMS time. For a number of years all went well until one afternoon, during a particularly severe episode of PMS, when her boss called her to his office to discuss a particular project. On the way to his office she was feeling very hostile, depressed and angry. She entered the meeting trying to control herself and her feelings, but suddenly and for no apparent reason, she started crying uncontrollably. She told her boss that he was an ass and he should take her job and stick it in his ear. "I quit," she yelled as she left the room. She immediately drove to our office and, in tears, told us what had happened.

Fortunately we were able to help her control her symptoms immediately. We encouraged her to go back to her boss and explain what had happened. We advised her to tell him the truth that she was experiencing PMS and that she has just started treatment for this condition. We suggested that she ask him to ignore her "resignation" and consider it as a plea for help. He did and her job was reinstated.

PMS AND ITS INFINITE VARIETY

The symptoms of PMS not only vary in severity, timing, duration and symptoms, but on occasion there may occur an aura, signaling the approaching onset of PMS symptoms, this is often more noticeable or worse in women with severe PMS or when PMS symptoms include migraine headaches. It is also common for there to be an increased level of activity prior to the onset of symptoms. During this time some woman may be driven to activities such as cleaning their house, shopping, exercising to excess, and they will often find themselves functioning with having had little sleep, and yet feeling euphoric. Some time later this increased level of activity is then followed by the onset of PMS symptoms, then fatigue, exhaustion, depression and a general inability to function. Occasionally, in some PMS women, migraine headaches may occur. When in some women they feel, "out of control," at this may soon herald the onset of symptoms of depression.

> ### PMS: Variations Over Time
>
> - **The symptoms of PMS can vary in type, duration and severity from day to day.**
> - **The symptoms of PMS can vary in type, duration and severity form month to month.**
> - **The symptoms of PMS can vary in type, duration and severity form year to year.**

Making the diagnosis of PMS depends not just on the symptoms manifested, nor the woman's predisposition toward PMS, nor their type or severity, but on their timing and their relationship to all of these other factors. When making the diagnosis of PMS, it is crucial to determine whether the symptoms are cyclic in nature; that is they exist in relationship to a woman's hormonal cycle. That is, they must occur within the week to two weeks prior to the onset of menstruation, the so-called Luteal Phase. While PMS usually is thought of only in relation to menstruating women, even a woman who has had her uterus removed (a hysterectomy), but still has at least one ovary can have PMS.

SUMMARY

PMS is a hormonal problem caused by a nutritional deficiency and worsened by an excess of "offender foods." It occurs in as many as 40% to 60% of all women. The symptoms are most commonly noticed by age 25 to 35. There are four groups of symptoms: the anxiety group, the hydrous or fluid group, the cravings group, and the depression group. PMS is most easily recognized by its symptom patterns related to the menstrual cycle. The most important diagnostic features are the recurrence of specific symptoms in the week to two weeks prior to the onset of menstruation (the luteal phase) and their disappearance with the onset of menstruation or shortly thereafter.

The most common symptoms of PMS are: cravings for sweets, swelling, bloating, irritability, lethargy and depression. In most women the period of time from normal menstrual bleeding to just prior to ovulation is generally symptom free. Symptoms occurring during this time cannot be attributed to PMS.

(This Page Is Purposefully Left Blank For You To Use To Take Notes)

CHAPTER 2

WHAT CAUSES PREMENSTRUAL SYNDROME?

While looking for a solution to Lisa's PMS problems we spent a number of months reading and evaluating all the information we could find about PMS. At that point in time the available information was quite confusing. First, we could find no clear cut agreement between any of the authors as to the exact cause of PMS. Next, we couldn't find a single method of treatment upon which they all agreed. And this hasn't changed much over the years.

During that period the majority of the literature on PMS was written by two researchers: Dr. Katherina Dalton, an English physician, and Dr. Guy Abraham, an OB-Gyn Endocrinologists at UCLA. Within a short time we had the opportunity to meet both of these magnificent people. We were especially fortunate to be able, subsequently, to study and work with Guy Abraham for the better part of a year.

Dr. Abraham's interest in PMS evolved during the early 1970's while he was researching a new biochemical testing procedure for evaluation of blood estrogen levels. During the course of this research he noticed that the estrogen levels of some of the women seemed to be higher than normal. He later recognized this group as women who had PMS. Eventually, he inferred that PMS was caused by an *excess of circulating estrogen*.

During the late 1950's, Dr. Dalton suggested that PMS was caused by *diminished levels of the female hormone progesterone*. She had worked with groups of women in England treating them with progesterone in the form of rectal and vaginal suppositories. She had each woman chart her pattern of symptoms before and after the onset of treatment. Her work clearly demonstrated that for a large proportion of the women treated with progesterone, PMS symptoms were relieved. Later she suggested, that in addition to natural progesterone therapy, PMS women should consume frequent small meals throughout the day. According to Dr. Dalton, this is useful for controlling many of the symptoms of PMS. She believed these small meals helped to stabilize the woman's blood sugar by keeping it from fluctuating uncontrollably during the day.

Through the process of our research into PMS we concluded that PMS is caused by an imbalance of two female hormones, *estrogen* and *progesterone*. In a sense both Dalton and Abraham are right. Whether one considers PMS to be caused by a decrease in progesterone or an increase in estrogen, depends entirely upon the direction from which you are looking at the imbalance. It's similar to the old question, "is the cup half empty or half full?"

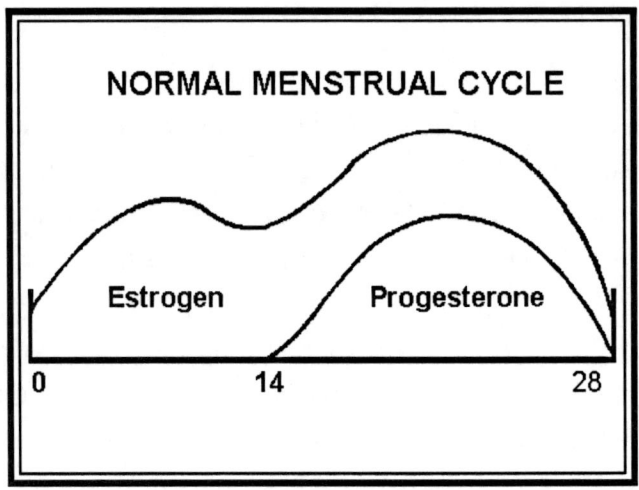

Figure A

We soon deduced from our work with our patients that PMS is caused by an alteration in the relationship between estrogen and progesterone, or better still, the *ratio of estrogen* to *progesterone*. That is, as estrogen rises, progesterone appears to fall, and vice versa. This is clearly demonstrated in Figures A & B.

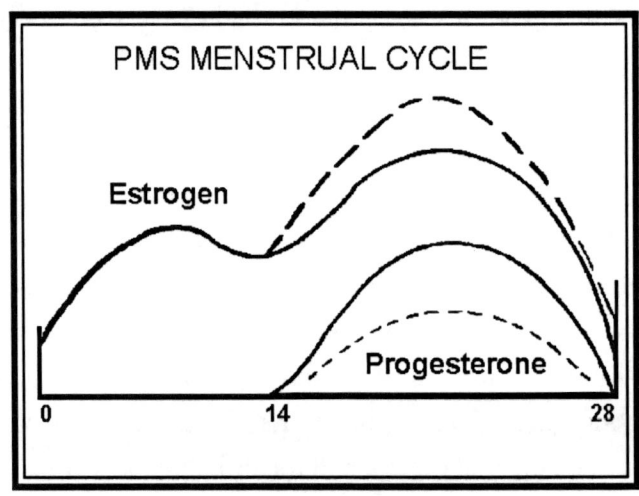

Figure B

In 1941 Dr. M. S. Biskins and his research group had noted that the human liver could not adequately break down and metabolize estrogen, unless it had a sufficient amount of B vitamins. From this Dr. Abraham postulated that both vitamin B6 (also known a pyridoxine or pyridoxine hydrochloride) and magnesium were needed to convert active circulating estrogen into its inactive *conjugated estrogen* form. This conversion is essential for controlling the level of circulating estrogen. Both magnesium and B vitamin's are required for the metabolism of amino acids, carbohydrates (especially refined sugars), and blood and tissue fats (lipids). The active forms of vitamin B6 is a necessary coenzyme for the transformation of DOPA to dopamine which will be discussed later one in the medical treatment section, where serotonin reuptake medications are discussed as a form of treatment for PMS. Vitamin B6 deficiency is also associated with elevated levels of Prolactin (also discussed in greater depth in the medical treatment section) and low levels of serotonin and dopamine. A deficiency of vitamin B6 can lead to depression, peripheral neuropathy (nerve injury), and mood changes.

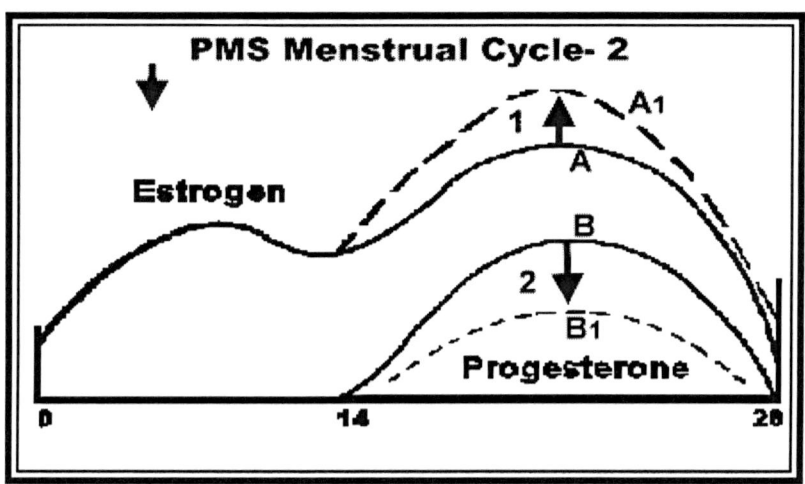

Figure C

As the level of estrogen rises (from A to A$_1$), whether there is any change in the level of progesterone or not, there is a change in the relationship between the levels of estrogen and progesterone. In other words as estrogen rises it can almost look as if the level of progesterone is decreasing even when it stays the same. The same is true in the oppositive direction, if estrogen stays the same but progesterone levels fall (from B to B$_1$) there is a change in the relationship or ratio of estrogen to progesterone. It is this change in the relationship or ratio between estrogen and progesterone that is the main cause for PMS. Each woman has her own personal ratio and when this ratio changes not only does it cause PMS symptoms, but it is also a sign that something is wrong. In the case of PMS that there are not sufficient essential nutrients to hold the estrogen levels in a normal ratio with progesterone, hence PMS is a symptom of a larger problem, a vitamin-mineral imbalance caused by too little magnesium and B6 reaching the woman's system and too much calcium and sugar in the diet.

In its inactive conjugated form, estrogen is more easily filtered and extracted by the kidneys and then eliminated. Without sufficient amounts of vitamin B6 and magnesium in the diet, the liver cannot transform the hormonally active estrogen into its conjugated form. This then causes the level of hormonally active estrogen circulating in the bloodstream to rise, creating an excess of active estrogen. As the levels of estrogen rise the woman develops an ever increasing propensity to PMS. Estrogen among its many effects in the female body can induce retention of salt and lower blood sugar, which as you read farther on, is responsible for a good

portion of the symptoms we think of as PMS symptoms. Once the estrogen-progesterone ratio reaches a critical level, where the ratio of estrogen to progesterone is abnormal enough, PMS symptoms develop. This phenomenon is demonstrated in Figures B, C, D and E.

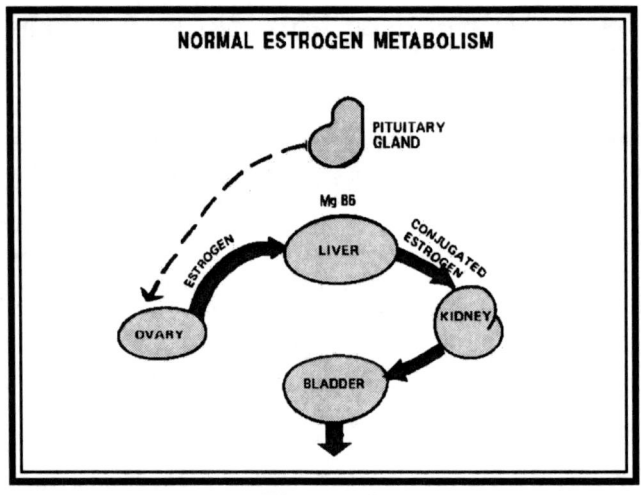

Figure D

This information clearly indicates that PMS is simply a symptom of a greater nutritional deficiency syndrome. Recognition of the role vitamin B6 and magnesium play in PMS suggested that there would be an advantage to be gained by increasing the dietary intake or supplementation of these essential substances.

To support this Dr. Abraham soon demonstrated clinically that PMS was improved and even eliminated by dietary modifications and supplements. Later, U. S. Department of
Agriculture studies produced evidence which would, indirectly, confirm this conclusion.

The U. S. Department of Agriculture studies indicated that some 40% of Americans have diets deficient in both vitamin B6 and magnesium. This correlates extremely well with the general incidence of PMS in American women. Our experience over the past 20 years demonstrates to us that PMS is indeed a nutritional deficiency syndrome which causes an imbalance of the female hormones estrogen and progesterone.

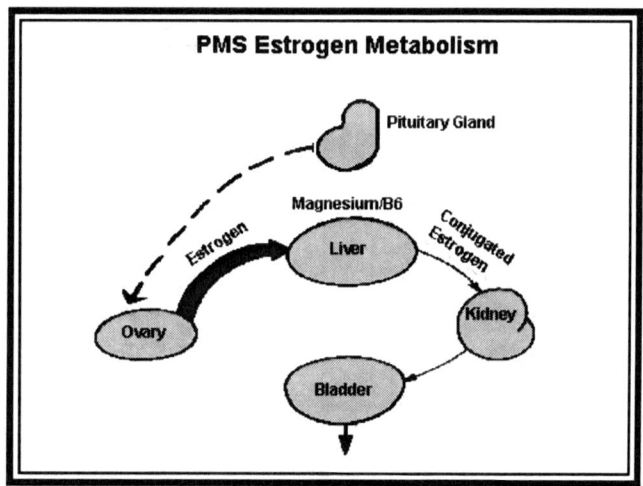

Figure E

Because of a deficiency of magnesium and/or vitamin B6 estrogen cannot be converted into its conjugated form, hence backs up into the woman's system.

A number of researchers have criticized the role of magnesium in creating PMS as Abraham had suggested, they use studies which demonstrate that serum levels of magnesium are often normal in women with PMS. However other researchers have clearly demonstrated that magnesium levels are definitely significantly lower within the red blood cells of with PMS suggesting that while magnesium levels are normal in the PMS woman's plasma, they are lower in her red blood cells hence less total magnesium is present and available for use by the woman's body, this therefore confirms Abraham's hypothesis. The role of calcium and dairy products and refined sugars in creating PMS, as indicated by Abraham are also confirmed as calcium interferes with the absorption of magnesium from the diet, and refined sugar increases the level of excretion (removal) of magnesium in the urine. To further support the role of magnesium deficiency in creating the symptoms of PMS we find that a magnesium deficiency can reduce dopamine and thyroid activity, which then contribute to an increase in the production and circulating levels of prolactin, which then can lead to depression, mood changes, and muscle cramping, some of the more common symptoms associated with PMS.

At this point, it is important to stress, and it will be stressed over and over again in this book, that each woman is an individual and if you try to apply one set of normals to all women you will find that you can make no headway with PMS. The imbalance in the estrogen- progesterone ratio is unique to each individual woman and is unlikely to be found nor defined by any of the present testing procedures used for determining estrogen or progesterone levels currently in use.

HOW DOES ONE BECOME DEFICIENT IN MAGNESIUM OR VITAMIN B6?

There are at least two ways in which a woman can become deficient in any vitamin or mineral:

1. **Absolute Deficiency:** This occurs when an individual's diet is either completely devoid of magnesium and/or vitamin B6 or lacks sufficient amounts of them to provide for all of the body's needs.

2. **Relative Deficiency:** There may be sufficient vitamin B6 and/or magnesium in your everyday diet, but there may also an excess of other foods in the diet which either inactivate them, compete with them or use them up. Excessive stress may also require increased levels of both magnesium and vitamin B6. These tend to create a situation which leaves the individual with insufficient nutrients to properly process her estrogen. Foods such as simple carbohydrates (sugar, honey, alcohol, processed foods), calcium rich foods (dairy or other foods high in calcium, or supplements high in calcium) and caffeine rich foods and beverages can do this. This is discussed in greater depth in the next chapter.

OTHER THEORIES REGARDING THE CAUSE OF PMS

While we are convinced through our own work as to the cause of PMS, the medical profession, requiring absolute proof before assigning a reason or cause to PMS, is not. To date many different theories have been offered regarding other possible causes for PMS. For completeness sake we will present some of the more reasonably accepted theories.

PROGESTERONE DEFICIENCY VERSES ABNORMAL PROGESTERONE THEORY

As we suggested earlier Dalton believed that PMS was due to a deficiency of progesterone. In our discussion above we suggested that we believed the most logical cause of PMS was an imbalance of the personal relationship or ratio between the PMS woman's own estrogen and her progesterone. Therefore correcting this imbalance should resolve the PMS problem. A J Rapkin, a well-respected PMS researcher, suggests that the problem may be an alteration in the brain response to normal progesterone ups and downs during the month and especially during the luteal phase. Rapkin suggests that the problem aries from a deficiency of allopregnanolone which is a psychoactive breakdown product of progesterone that has specific effect in the brain and central nervous system.

Allopregnanolone and pregnenolone, two breakdown products of progesterone, are both individually referred to as *neurosteroids*. They interact with the gamma-aminobutyric acid A also known as GABA-A which is receptor complex. These neurosteroids can alter the excitability of brain neurons through their interaction with other neurotransmitter. Rapkin's data suggests allopregnanolone enhances GABA-A receptor function and acts to reduce anxiety. Therefore, a deficiency in this neurosteroid might predispose to anxiety in the face of almost any challenge. Pregnenolone, on the other hand, may antagonize GABA-A receptors and promote anxiety. Thus perhaps brain cells, in women with PMS, breakdown progesterone secreted by the ovary into pregnenolone rather than into allopregnanolone hence ending up not only deprived of the anxiety reducing neurosteroid, but they might also be exposed to higher concentrations of a neurosteroid that increases anxiety. While this is still not completely proven, it can help us to further understand the role of progesterone in creating PMS.

PROLACTIN THEORY

Prolactin, a hormone made by the anterior pituitary, causes the stimulation of breast-milk production after childbirth. It is intimately tied in with the levels of both estrogen and progesterone. It has long been known that prolactin levels reach their peak around the time of ovulation and then remain elevated during the post ovulation into the luteal phase, the exact timing is quite consistent with the time when PMS occurs. When prolactin is produced in excessive amounts, it is often associated with irregular menstruation, decreased interest in sex, depression, and increased levels of hostility. These are relatively common symptoms often found in women with PMS. It is also presumed that prolactin plays a role in the over-stimulation of the breast which may be related to premenstrual breast tenderness, another symptom found commonly in PMS. The problem with this theory is that there have been no consistent abnormalities of prolactin levels found in women with PMS. Therefore, it cannot be tied directly to PMS as a primary cause. On its own elevations of prolactin levels are rare and while it may be associated with some symptoms of PMS, one rarely sees the onset of full-blown premenstrual syndrome in women who have elevated prolactin levels.

This also leads us to another problem, it does not account for all of the 90 or more other symptoms that are not related to any symptoms to elevated prolactin, but which are found in true PMS. The possibility however, does exist that since the circulating levels of both estrogen and progesterone are both directly and indirectly related to production of prolactin and its circulating levels that it may be part of a more generalized imbalance between estrogen and progesterone. Therefore when estrogen and progesterone are thrown out of balance, this may ultimately relate to an imbalance of prolactin and possibly an imbalance between prolactin and estrogen and prolactin and progesterone, as well as an imbalance between prolactin and the estrogen-progesterone ratio. This might suggest the possibility that prolactin does play a role, even if it is an indirect role, in the creation of PMS and certain PMS symptoms.

ALDOSTERONE THEORY

Aldosterone is a hormone made by the adrenal glands, its primary role is to help maintain blood pressure by causing your kidneys to retain salt (sodium) and eliminate potassium. When too much sodium is retained then water is also retained and blood pressure goes up. It has been noticed that aldosterone levels normally increase around the time of ovulation and they remain elevated during the week to two weeks before the onset of menstruation. Once again this is consistent with the timing of PMS. It is theorized that this elevation of aldosterone that might be responsible for the PMS-H or congestive symptoms of PMS such as edema, breast swelling, abdominal bloating, weight gain, and headaches. Once again, however, there are little or no consistent differences in the total circulating levels of aldosterone between PMS women and non-PMS women when both are studied. What role, if any, aldosterone plays in the creation of or maintenance of PMS is still unclear. If it is related, it is likely either a contributing member of the generalized hormonal imbalance which may be triggered by the abnormal ratio of estrogen to progesterone or a pawn in whatever causes this imbalance, likely once again a nutritional imbalance.

THE ENDORPHIN THEORY

Some researchers have noticed that there is an increased level of certain endorphins, specifically, beta-endorphins, after ovulation. Endorphins are opiate-like neuro-chemicals made by the woman's brain and her body to reduce pain and induce an increased sense of well-being. These researchers have suggested that women with PMS may produce fewer endorphins or suffer from a more sudden withdrawal from their activity and therefore these women are more likely to experience increased sensitivity to pain and depression during the week to two weeks prior to the onset of their menses, the time PMS is more likely to occur, the luteal phase.

The main problem with this theory is that once again the results of testing levels of beta-endorphins during the menstrual cycle are mixed and ultimately considered inconclusive. No consistent pattern of decreased beta-endorphin levels has ever been noted in the week to two weeks after ovulation nor prior to the onset of menstruation.

HYPOGLYCEMIA OR LOW BLOOD SUGAR THEORY

The woman's body appears to be more sensitive to insulin during her luteal phase. This information has lead PMS researchers to theorize that short-lived episodes of low blood sugar (hypoglycemia) caused by this increased amount of insulin breaking down circulating blood sugar may account for some PMS symptoms. Once again hypoglycemia and increased insulin production as well as insulin release is commonly seen in response to a diet which is high in refined sugars and since insulin production and utilization is closely related to availability of magnesium, it is clear that this theory of PMS is quite consistent with the dietary deficiency-excess theory which we subscribe to. The hypoglycemia theory can lead directly a number of the more important PMS symptoms including fatigue, racing heart, sugar craving (both as cause and result), mood swings, difficulty concentrating, feelings of anxiety, food cravings, addictions and binging, to name only the more important ones.

PROSTAGLANDINS

Prostaglandins are a group of hormone-like substances which play a role in a wide variety of internal chemical processes yet act differently in different tissues of the body. They play a role in such areas as arthritis and rheumatism, fighting inflamation and infection, vascular constriction, the movement of calcium in and out of cells, the regulation of certain hormones and cell growth control.

Prostaglandins are also associated with breast pain, fluid retention, abdominal cramping, headaches, irritability, and depression. Physical premenstrual complaints and painful menstruation have been shown to respond positively to prostaglandin inhibitors. These chemicals act to either decrease the formation of prostaglandins or block its affects. The most common and easiest available products in this group are non-steroidal anti-inflammatory (NSAID's) medications.

Once again you can immediately see an interrelationship between prostaglandins and calcium which then means that there is also an effect relating to magnesium, since calcium and magnesium always affect each other, prostaglandins will likely also be at the effect of dietary calcium and magnesium levels.

STRESS

One of the many theories of PMS is that it is both directly and indirectly related to stress. Initially this does not sound outrageous as so many of the symptoms of PMS are also symptoms of stress or are symptoms of effects caused by stress, for example, anxiety, depression, irritability, food cravings, headaches etc., however, so many other symptoms cannot such as edema, swelling, and others cannot be explained by stress alone.

If one broadens the concept to suggest that chronic recurrent episodes of stress can so unbalance the body, interfere with the endocrine system and create nutritional deficiencies and hormonal imbalances then stress could definitely be considered as a primary cause of PMS. However, while this can happen it is unlikely to be the sole cause or etiology of PMS

PSYCHOSOCIAL THEORY

Emotional and physical stressors have been found to influence the menstrual cycle. Travel, illness, stress, weather changes, and other environmental factors may affect ovulation, length of menstrual cycle, and severity of PMS. Cultural attitudes, the attitudes of society, as well as personal attitudes toward menstruation and PMS also appear to play a role in the presence and severity of PMS. The dynamic interplay of our environment, spirit, and physiology demands an integrated medical-psychosocial approach to the treatment of PMS. Many women appear to have learned to have PMS symptoms from their mother's, sister's and other relatives, family and friends. We have known this for years and when we work with each woman on an individual basis we always must be aware of the role her family, spouses (past and present), her lifestyle, dietary choices, work, career, life stresses and spiritual conflicts play to reduce pressure on the woman. We also look for whatever role these factors play in both the creation and severity of her PMS.

INDIVIDUAL AND CULTURAL ATTITUDES

There has been suggestion that both the beliefs of the individual woman and those of the specific culture that she comes from play a role in the creation, experiencing and severity of PMS symptoms. Within this context it is believed that a primary factor is the woman's attitudes and beliefs regarding menstruation. The prevailing theory is that PMS goes along with a generally negative attitude toward menstruation. Studies have suggested that women who have more positive attitudes regarding menstruation tend to have fewer problems with PMS. Others believe that some stereo-typed beliefs, for example, about menstruation have over the centuries contributed to how PMS symptoms are experienced.

As couples, males and females clearly appear to influence each other in regards to attitude, levels of awareness of menstruation and aggressivity and the roles of males and females in any society. In 1989 Abraham & Mira studied couples and relationships and found that the onset of personal relationship problems often occurred about the same time as the development of PMS symptoms. It has also been found that the woman's social health and lack of strength of her supportive systems more significantly contribute to her PMS experience than either stress or her physical health and well-being. As we have said earlier under contributing factors, marital status is a major contributor toward PMS.

The question also runs the other way as PMS is often seen as an excuse women can use to get out of work, from taking care of home, and maintain power over men. Still others suggest that PMS is a conspiracy against women in that PMS may be a way for women to express their aggressiveness, others believe that by society telling them that something is wrong with PMS, this makes women appear more negatively aggressive and that this is wrong, hence PMS symptoms are a reaction against this. Therefore, if society picks up on female emotions (especially to those considered negative by men or by society itself) and constantly relates them to menstruation, then Premenstrual

Syndrome is a likely outcome. Finally, PMS has been seen by some as a reflection of male dominance. This then suggests that the female self-image must clearly be a reflection of the patriarchal view point in western culture.

The ultimate role of attitudes, by the PMS sufferer, other women, the society, men, the social structure in the creation or worsening of PMS still is unclear and needs much more thought and work to determine what is what and how each affects the other.

In another set of challenging statistics regarding women who suffer from PMS, it was found in one study performed looking at women with severe PMS, that at least 95% of the women in this study suffered at least one attempted or completed act of sexual abuse. Of these women 81% reported complete penetration against their will, and 85% of the women stated that they sustained physical threat or actual injury. When this is compared to other studies of sexually abused women in general populations, it was determined that PMS women were abused earlier in life, more frequently, and by similar types of offenders.

Of the women who had reported having been abused, 65% were found to also suffer from post-traumatic stress disorder (PTSD). Most these abused women, 83% had up to the time of the study, never disclosed that they had been abuse to any of their prior health practitioners. The conclusion of this study suggested that a history of sexual abuse, particularly during childhood or adolescence, may be extremely common among women seeking treatment for severe PMS, and that substantial undiagnosed PTSD may also be present in this group.

Since the majority of these women had never talked about the abuse they suffered or let any physician help them, most received little or no emotional or psychological help for the trauma they had experienced. The majority of these women carried their emotional and psychological scars around with them well into their later years.

CHAPTER SUMMARY

No matter which theory of the cause of PMS you chose to believe in it soon becomes clear that diet, and specifically excesses of refined and processed foods and calcium, along with the resultant deficiency of magnesium and vitamin B6 and other very essential vitamins, minerals, fatty acids and nutrients play an important role in the creation of PMS. However, while this may be a primary cause, it is often not the only factor which finally determines which symptoms are most likely going to occur, nor how sever these symptoms are ultimately going to be.

In the end just about all of the various theories presented above can be fit into or can connect up with dietary excess and deficiencies and can often be explained as a consequence of these excesses and deficiencies.

(This Page Is Purposefully Left Blank For You To Use To Take Notes)

CHAPTER 3

PMS TREATMENTS AND TREATMENT STRATEGIES

INTRODUCTION

All through the long history of Western medicine, the specific medical treatment program used to treat a medical condition has generally been based on the existing belief of the time as to the cause of the illness or condition. The same is true of PMS, today's physician will likely base his or her choice of a treatment program on what he or she believes is the most correct theory for the cause of PMS. Since as we have already suggested that there is no one cause or reason for PMS which has been accepted by the medical profession, the choice of treatment will most likely vary from doctor to doctor and will likely be based on the personal opinion as to what the "real" reason for PMS is.

The specific form of treatment used for any woman will depend on two noteworthy considerations. First, who chooses the method of treatment, the PMS woman or her doctor, and secondly, how much both know about PMS and the various methods that are used to treat it.

This means that if your doctor agrees with us that PMS is a nutritional disorder, than he or she might either suggest a nutritional approach, that is, refilling deficiencies using a diet rich in essential nutrients to undo deficiencies and eliminate excesses, or if on the other hand, if your doctor is primarily medically oriented he or she may choose to treat this same imbalance of estrogen and progesterone with a more traditional Western medical form of therapy to attack the production of estrogen and progesterone directly with either medication or surgery. If your practitioner is oriented to Eastern medicine, he or she might suggest that your PMS be treated with herbs, acupuncture, acupressure or body-energy work

30 Days To No More PMS

SUMMARY OF APPROACHES TO THE TREATMENT OF PMS

Presently there are three categories of treatment commonly used to deal with PMS:

1. Medical Treatments for PMS
   a. Hormonal Approach
      i.   Oral Contraceptives
      ii. Ovarian Suppression
      iii. Gonadotropin-Releasing Hormone Agonist (GnRH-A)
   b. Diuretics
   c. Tranquilizers, Mood Elevators and Pain Killers
   d. Serotonin Reuptake Inhibitors
   e. Anti-inflammatory Medications
2. A Nutritional Approach
   a. General Dietary Measures
   b. Magnesium and Calcium
   c. Vitamin B6
   d. Vitamin E
3. Other Non-Traditional Medical Approaches
   a. Exercise
   b. Primrose Oil
   c. Herbal and Botanical Medicines
   d. Acupuncture
   e. Acupressure
   f. Body-Energy work
4. A Combined Approach, Elements of Two or More of the Above Approaches

MEDICAL TREATMENTS FOR PMS

The Hormonal Approach To Treating PMS

The Hormonal Approach is usually associated with the concept that PMS is caused either by a *deficiency of progesterone* or an *excess of estrogen*. The ultimate goal of hormonal therapy may vary with who administers it. In one approach, progesterone levels are artificially raised to reestablish the progesterone-estrogen ratio. In another approach, estrogen levels are suppressed. In still another approach ovulation is blocked hence controlling both estrogen and progesterone production. In the following section we will discuss the current approaches and how they are used, their effectiveness, benefits and the problems associated with them.

Treating With Natural Progesterone

As we stated earlier, Dr. Dalton began treating PMS women with natural progesterone in the mid 1950's. Natural progesterone is used to raise the blood progesterone levels to normalize the balance between estrogen and progesterone as seen in Figures B and C above.

Under Dr. Dalton's guidance, natural progesterone became the first successful treatment of PMS. Today thousands of women all over the world are being helped by the use of this method. Natural progesterone presently can be taken in the form of rectal or vaginal suppositories and fluids or intra-muscular injection. Some pharmacies in the United States are making an orally active form. However, this form has not been approved by the Food and Drug Administration (FDA) as of the publication of our 30-Days to No More PMS program.

As we have previously suggested, the main downfall with so many of the treatments for PMS is that they do not treat the underlying cause of PMS. It is a nutritional-dietary imbalance that has caused the imbalance in the estrogen-progesterone ratio. While it may re-approximate the estrogen/progesterone to a more normal-appearing level and hence eliminate the symptoms of PMS, it does not solve the cause of PMS. It does however, in many PMS women reduce or even eliminate their symptoms and make life much better for them.

Natural, or better still, Bio-Identical Progesterone in the form of vaginal and rectal suppositories, vaginal pessaries, pellets implanted under the skin, and injections must be used in doses sufficient to relieve PMS symptoms. They must be prescribed by a medical doctor or nurse practitioner and close follow-up is required. This method has problems in that some women experience a recurrence of symptoms after one to six months of therapy (again since the underlying cause has not been dealt with). An increase in the dosage is then necessary until a new level of relief is established. More than 50% of women using one or another form of progesterone complain of side effects or adverse reactions including menstrual irregularities, irregular vaginal bleeding, headaches, and vaginal itching. It is often costly, messy and often very inconvenient. Oral micronized progesterone had fewer side effects, but also fewer positive results. In one study, it was concluded that oral micronized progesterone is ineffective in treating PMS.

Synthetic progesterones, or progestogens, in the form of Provera or oral contraceptives often worsen PMS symptoms. These synthetic hormones are generally 100 to 2,000 times more powerful than natural progesterone. Suppressing production of the woman's own progesterone, they may prolong PMS symptoms from weeks to months. Their use should be avoided in PMS women.

Oral Contraceptives

Earlier we discussed oral contraceptives as a potential problem in creating PMS, on the other hand, if subscribe to the theory that PMS is caused by an imbalance of estrogen and progesterone, either as a primary mechanism or as a secondary cause, then creating a stable relationship or ratio between circulating estrogen and progesterone would immediately seem like a reasonable approach to treating PMS. Birth control pills are used because they contain a measured amount of both estrogens and progestogens, therefore can, it is often believed can correct the estrogen-progesterone imbalance. Another specific logic for using oral contraceptives is that they act to suppress ovulation and therefore eliminate the luteal phase and because of this they eliminate PMS.

In fact, in some women birth control pills do work to eliminate or at least reduce PMS symptoms. Unfortunately, this does not happen in all women. In some BCP's may make PMS symptoms much worse. The reason why it does work in some women, but not all women is simple, but not always apparent to many physicians. The problem in PMS, is not simply that there is too much estrogen and too little progesterone, but rather that there is an imbalance in the relationship or ratio between these two hormones. This ratio is specific to each individual woman and a ratio that is perfect for one woman might be a major problem, causing PMS, for another woman. Her personal ratio is part of her uniqueness as an individual woman. When you, as medicine generally does, try to fit all women (or men) into a single one-answer fits all mold, you cannot do this. The end result of why one woman placed on a specific birth control pill will do perfectly well, and another will not, appears to relate almost entirely to the specific type of hormone used and the relationship of its strength, potency and dosage. If, after going on BCP's, her estrogen-progesterone ratio ends up in a range similar to her normal range, then her symptoms will go away. If the estrogen-progesterone ratio ends up either decreased or increased, out of her normal range then her symptoms may become significantly worse. What works for one may not work for another. Sometimes simply trying different pill combinations might allow you to find one that works, but this can be costly, time consuming and potentially a problem as symptoms might get worse before and if they ever get better.

Unfortunately, the use of oral contraceptives for ovarian suppression has many problems. The most important problem is that many women will develop virtually continuous PMS symptoms while on specific birth control pills. Others have a rebound reaction in which their original PMS symptoms significantly worsen when they finally discontinue the birth control pills. As we discussed earlier, oral contraceptives are made with *synthetic progestogens* (often also called *progestins*) which suppress the woman's own *natural progesterone* production hence even further lowering her circulating progesterone and throwing her estrogen-progesterone ratio off that much further. These progestogens can stimulate a worsening of PMS symptoms in many women. And often the resulting symptoms are much worse than they were originally.

When a specific woman needs contraception, wants to take the pill and it also works to reduce or eliminate her PMS symptoms, then everyone is usually happy and we have a success story. On the other hand, when a specific woman uses birth control pills and her symptoms worsen, she should stop these pills, either try another combination, or use a totally different method for contraception, and another method for treatment of her PMS.

Recent studies evaluating a relatively new contraceptive pill appear to be quite hopeful. The pill is called, Yasmin. It contains a new type of hormone which may effectively treat PMS symptoms. This new hormone is called Drospirenone. Drospirenone is a progestin and it is believed to have diuretic properties because it is similar in structure to a water pill called spironolactone. While it is not yet approved for the treatment of PMS, many doctors and women, are already choosing it as their contraceptive of choice because of its ability to reduce PMS symptoms.

In the manufacturer-funded study, more than 800 women who were given Yasmin were later surveyed about their PMS symptoms. Nearly 72% of the women in the study reported that they had suffered from PMS. During the month before entry into the study, half of the women reported that they were either treating themselves or being treated for their symptoms with either over-the-counter PMS medications, prescription or alternative medications.

Before to starting this new oral contraceptive, 30% of the women reported that PMS affected their daily activities, however this figure dropped to 16% for those on the pill. The number of women reporting that PMS affected their general well-being also dropped, from 35% prior to taking the birth control pill to 21% while on it.

Researchers noticed positive effects regarding reduction of weight gain, breast swelling, anxiety, restlessness, food cravings, irritability, depression, and other symptoms of PMS, were reported for both women who had not taken oral contraceptives prior to taking Yasmin and for those women who switched to Yasmin from another birth control pill.

While this study is far from decisive, critics suggest that ultimate outcome of the study in regard to PMS could have easily been influenced by the fact that the women most likely had been told Yasmin might relieve their PMS symptoms. Once critic stated in regard to this study, "You certainly can't rule out the placebo effect here, but it is interesting that even women who had used another form of oral contraceptive reported a very positive experience with the drospirenone-containing pill." Studies are currently under way to determine if Yasmin is effective against the most severe form of PMS, known as premenstrual dysphoric disorder (PMDD).

The use of oral contraceptive, birth control pills, are contraindicated in any woman who is a smoker or have had a prior problem with deep venous thrombophlebitis, pulmonary embolus, or thrombosis.

Once again we feel it is important to note that while BCP's work, using them does not correct the underlying cause nor the long term risks associated with their deficiencies.

Suppression of Ovulation

Many years ago physicians noted that PMS "went away" during pregnancy. In recent years, a number of medical treatments have been based on the notion of creating a pseudo state of pregnancy through the suppression of ovarian function can eliminate PMS symptoms. Oral contraceptives (birth control pills) have been used for many years for this purpose. More recently, several medications, the best known of which is Danazol, have also been used for this purpose. Danazol is used particularly when the PMS symptoms are severe and "nothing else seems to work."

Danazol appears to work using a slightly different mechanism then BCP's. It is not a progestogen but rather acts to suppress the hypothalamic-pituitary-ovarian axis (See Diagrams A-D) thereby suppressing estrogen production and altering the metabolism of the sexual hormones. It has a weak androgenic (male) hormonal affect as well. Danazol, known under the brand name of Danocrine, is not specifically recommended for the treatment of PMS. It is recommended for treatment of a number of the conditions which are high-estrogen problems such as endometriosis, fibrocystic disease of the breasts and hormonal conditions which cause pain in one or both breasts.

Danazol is not specifically approved by the Food and Drug Administration for the treatment of PMS and little or no research has been done to approve its efficacy in PMS. Danazol is approved only for short periods of use -- 6 to 9 months, at most. For many women, Danazol also has a number of side effects which can be quite disconcerting. For example: weight gain, fluid retention, acne, and seborrhea (dandruff). These, however, are generally temporary and fully reversible. Other side effects such as mild hirsutism (growth of facial and body hair), swelling, hair loss, voice changes (hoarseness), and sore throat are not necessarily reversible and may persist after treatment is discontinued. Menstrual cycles are often stopped and occasionally continuous vaginal bleeding or spotting can occur. These side affects are generally accounted for by its androgenic (male hormone) effects.

The major problem with Danazol, however, is that its effects on PMS are primarily limited to the time in which the woman is using it. Occasionally some women will get long-standing results, but PMS frequently returns at some point in the future either unabated or even worsened. On the other hand, when PMS is suppressed for any length of time, one perplexing after effect that occurs relatively frequently is that some women may not menstruate for months or even years after this therapy. In some case's pregnancy is impossible for a period of time after completion of even a short term of treatment. Finally, once again the real cause of PMS is not being treated.

Treatment of PMS With Gonadotropin-Releasing Hormone Agonist (GnRH-A)

In recent years many physicians have been using Gonadotropin-Releasing Hormone Agonist often simply refer to as GnRH-A's to treat PMS. Once again the logic is to deal with the imbalance between estrogen and progesterone. The goal of using GnRH-A medications is to suppress the production of estrogen and progesterone, rather than to either raise progesterone levels or lower estrogen levels, nor to reestablish the most appropriate and normal estrogen-progesterone ratio for the individual woman. In the following sections we will look briefly at this form of treatment, its pros and cons and more about the logic behind its use. Since it is a relatively new treatment, we well go into greater depth about it than some of the other methods we have just discuss below.

There are a number of products that have been used to treat PMS. This includes Leuprolide acetate (sold as Lupron Depot, Injectable, Eligard and Viadur Implants), nafarelin acetate (Synarel Nasal

Spray) and goserelin acetate (Zoladex).

Leuprolide is given either as a daily, or once every 1 to 3 months intramuscular injection. Nafarelin is a nasal spray used twice a day and goserelin is injected into the fat tissue of the abdomen once every 28 days.

How Does Using GnRH-A Work To Prevent PMS?

Gonadotropin-releasing hormone agonist (GnRH-A) are medications which work at the level of the pituitary gland to suppress the production of Follicle-Stimulating Hormone (FSH – which stimulates the development of an egg each month prior to ovulation and the production of the female hormone estrogen) and Luteinizing Hormone (LH – which stimulates the development of a corpus luteum cyst in the ovary which produces the female hormone progesterone). The end result of using GnRH-A is a reduction in the amount of estrogen in the body, and prevention of ovulation (the release of eggs from the ovaries). These changes work to stop the monthly menstrual hormonal cycle and create an artificial state similar to menopause. The net result is no development of an egg, no estrogen, no menstruation, and no PMS.

What Is The Main Value In Using GnRH-A As A Treatment For PMS?

GnRH-A medications are generally used to prevent PMS symptoms, when all other medical treatments, including those which prevent ovulation, have failed.

GnRH-A's has been used as a kind of trial to see if PMS will occur one both ovaries (oophorectomy) have been removed to test whether or not the woman will then suffer from intractable PMS. If treatment with this medication is able to adequately relieve PMS symptoms, then the removal of both ovaries will likely provide her a complete relief from her PMS symptoms. Keep in mind, however, that even if her symptoms do improve with GnRH-A treatment, it is still possible that the medication was not the only reason for her improvement.

GnRH-A's should only be used for short periods of time (3 to 6 months) and generally no longer, therefore they generally only used as a stop gap before surgery is decided upon.

GnRH-A medications are often use in the management of conditions such as endometriosis, uterine fibroid tumors, increased hair growth (hirsutism), irregular or non-malignant uterine bleeding, and breast and prostate cancers. While used to treat PMS, GnRH-A's are not specifically approved for the treatment of PMS.

How Well Does GnRH-A Work?

These medications are quite potent and in most cases they will result in complete eliminations of the physical, emotional and psychological symptoms caused by PMS. The effectiveness of the nafarelin nasal spray can be hard to define.

In a number of research studies women with PMS who were placed on GnRH-A improved significantly when compared to women who were given placebos. The women who had PMS symptoms all through the month and had PMS-like symptoms in combination with dysphoric symptoms (that is suffering from pain, discomfort, depression, unhappiness, usually referred to as the PMS-D group) symptoms did not improve significantly, although specific symptoms such as irritability and depression did appear to improve to some degree. Women more frequently described themselves as more friendly and cheerful than usual, during their premenstrual period. Physical symptoms such as swelling and headache showed significant improvement. Breast tenderness however remained unaffected. True depressive symptoms improved in the PMS group, but not in the PMS-D group. It did however take several months of treatment with leuprolide before recognizable clinical results were seen. There was no evidence that PMS symptoms were worsened with treatment. These results repeat the findings of other studies suggesting that leuprolide reduced PMS symptoms to minimal levels when PMS symptoms occurred in the week to two weeks before the onset of menstruation. The fact that leuprolide was not effective in women with ongoing dysphoric symptoms, confirms our belief that premenstrual depression (PMS-D) may have an entirely different mechanisms of action than that of other dysphoric-depressive mood disorders that last all month long or come randomly during the month.

It should be understood that none of these medications are specifically approved for the treatment of PMS, rather they are used to test whether complete suppression of all female hormones will in fact "turn off" the mechanism that is causing PMS, elevated estrogen and decreased progesterone. Therefore they really do not treat the cause of PMS, but merely the symptoms of PMS.

What, If Any, Are The Side Effects of GnRH-A Medications?

GnRH-A medications produce a chemical menopause, with many, if not most, of the same symptoms and side effects of true menopause. Fortunately, these symptoms and side effects generally go away on their own when the GnRH-A medication is stopped.

- Absence of periods (amenorrhea)
- Absence of ovulation
- So-called a "medical oophorectomy," A chemical removal of the ovaries by suppression of FSH and LH.
- Hot flashes
- Mood swings
- Vaginal dryness
- Decreased sexual interest
- Loss of bone density
- Increased total cholesterol level
- Decreased high-density lipoprotein (HDL) cholesterol, hence increased risk of coronary artery disease
- Acne (with nafarelin use)
- Nasal irritation (with nafarelin use)
- Lower urinary tract symptoms (with goserelin use)

Besides these primary side effects there are a few less consistent, but still potential problems:

- They cannot be used in any women who desires becoming pregnant, for if pregnancy occurs while using these medications, severe fetal abnormalities or fetal death may occur.
- Liver dysfunction, along with abnormal liver function tests, may occur with use of leuprolide's.
- Increased hair growth may occur
- Headaches
- The risk of vaginal infection is increased
- Low blood pressure may occur
- Irregular vaginal bleeding or spotting may occur

With prolonged use, greater than 6 months, increased bone loss may lead to permanent loss of bone density and irreversible osteoporosis, and may increase the risk for bone fractures later in life. When used only for short periods of time, less than 6 months, its effects are probably reversible and generally will not become a major problem.

Women often become somewhat depressed or anxious when they first begin GnRH-A treatment.

Though you are not likely to become pregnant while taking this medication, studies have shown that GnRH-A medications may adversely affect a developing fetus. A reliable birth control method should be used during the entire time the woman is taking a GnRH-A medication.

Combined Therapy

The benefit's of GnRH-A appear to be increased even more, when it is used along with estrogen and a progestin in a combined treatment program. In such case, two things are likely to be happening: 1) Ovulation is suppressed by the GnRh-A and therefore the imbalance between estrogen and progesterone, which is causing the PMS is eliminated, and 2) the estrogen and progestin are being used in order to eliminate the menopause-like symptoms caused by the GnRH-A medication. When they are used in the usual therapeutic dosages, they will then secondarily act to further eliminate the estrogen-progesterone imbalance.

Other Issues to Think About

- GnRH-A treatment usually stops menstrual periods. If regular periods continue, this should be discussed with your doctor.
- GnRH-A treatment should be considered only after all other treatments for PMS have been tried.
- You should certainly to consider your risk for bone loss and osteoporosis before starting any program of long term GnRH-A therapy. If you are at high risk, you may want to consider a form of treatment.
- Because of the potential risk of osteoporosis, you will want to avoid repeating GnRH-A therapy. If a second course of GnRH-A treatment is needed, you will best wait at least one full year before starting it.

- GnRH-A treatment is quite costly, you should first consider the possible benefits to you and the effectiveness of this form of treatment, as well as compare side effects with other possible treatment programs.

Diuretics

As we suggested earlier elevated levels of estrogen can result in increased salt retention, because of this many physicians believe that a mild diuretic can be helpful in reducing the increased fluid, swelling and water retention created during the PMS period. Diuretics are therefore frequently used to treat the swelling and bloating associated with PMS. Even though their purpose is to alleviate swelling, they rarely affect the other symptoms and are no longer considered efficacious. We have found that swelling is related to the amount of sugar and calcium in the woman's diet and therefore control of the intake of these substances and the foods that contain them is a much better treatment. When these foods are appropriately controlled, the swelling ceases to be a problem. Increasing total water intake may also help.

Tranquilizers, Mood Elevators and Pain Killers

Another approach used to treating some of the symptoms of PMS, especially depression, mood swings, irritability, the PMS-a group symptoms, is with medications such as tranquilizers, antidepressants, mood elevators, sleeping pills, pain killers or other medications. These alter mood or change the PMS woman's ability to cope with her symptoms. Medications such as Valium, Xanax, Librium, Ativan, Codeine, Phenobarbital, Tranxene, Pamelor, Parnate, Prozac, Sinequan, Elavil, Triavil, Tofranil, Wellbutrin, Lithium, Thorazine, Haldol, Desoxyn, Ritalin, Cylert and many other similar types of medications have been used at one time or another to treat PMS women.

Very few women however ultimately report improvement on such regimes. Most feel misdirected or even dehumanized and their symptoms may even worsen. Just as women who have psychiatric problems can also experience PMS, women with PMS can experience severe emotional problems. Women who suffer PMS should never be considered to have psychiatric problems just because they have PMS. The symptoms of PMS are frequently misdiagnosed even by competent physicians when care is not taken to obtain a very thorough and directed medical and menstrual cycle history. For the less enlightened doctor, certain symptoms of PMS can certainly make it appear as if there is a psychiatric condition. If a woman is not educated about her PMS she may even fall victim to believing that she in fact does have a psychiatric problem.

Treating PMS as a psychiatric problem often delays correct treatment of the underlying hormonal imbalance and its causes. By allowing the nutritional deficiencies to go unrepaired, there is a worsening of the process, leaving the woman with no room for hope.

If a genuine psychiatric problem exists and either has triggered a worsening of PMS symptoms or is the cause of symptoms that have been linked to PMS or where wrongfully believed to be caused by PMS, this woman should be referred to a psychiatrist for appropriate diagnosis and treatment.

Selective Serotonin Reuptake Inhibitors

Selective serotonin reuptake inhibitors have been used for many years for treating depression, the thought was that since one of the more common symptoms of PMS is depression why not use serotonin reuptake inhibitors to treat PMS.

To this end a number of controlled studies were performed which showed that selective serotonin reuptake inhibitors (SSRI) are indeed effective for both severe PMS and PMDD. Fluoxetine (Prozac) 10 mg per day was put up against vitamin B6 (pyridoxine) 300 mg per day, 0.75 mg per day, and propanolol (Inderal) 20 mg and 40 mg per day. All were given only during the menstrual period. Results were as follows, fluoxetine reduced PMS symptoms by 65.4%, propanolol by 58.7%, pyridoxine by 45.3%; and placebo, by 39.4% to 46.1%. The authors of this study ultimately concluded that fluoxetine, 10 mg once daily, presented the best results for treating PMS.

A 1999 review concluded that fluoxetine 20 mg per day is an effective and well-tolerated treatment for women with PMDD. Paroxetine (Paxil, also a selective serotonin reuptake inhibitor) and sertraline (Zoloft, not a selective serotonin reuptake inhibitor) also appeared to have equal effectiveness. The selective serotonin reuptake inhibitors are superior to most other classes of antidepressants for the treatment of PMS symptoms.

When use of fluoxetine was compared to psychological treatment (cognitive therapy) alone or in combination, that is, fluoxetine and cognitive therapy combined. There was little or no differences, except that after 6 months, the therapy group was better off then the group which used fluoxetine alone.

Stress Management

Since stress can be a major contributor to the causes of PMS, this suggests that a stress management treatment program would be logical value in preventing or treating PMS. Unfortunately for most physicians this means treating their patients with anti-anxiety medications, tranquilizers to reduce anxiety in order to reduce the effect of stress on the individual. Tranquilizers however, really only cover up the reasons for stress and anxiety, they neither solve the underlying symptoms nor in the end do they really provide a helpful treatment of PMS. A true Stress management program without using medication is a much better choice.

The first step of the enlightened physician is to explain to his or her stressed patient the role of stress in creating PMS. While we are not going to get into the basic chemistry of stress and how it potentiates PMS in this book, we can point to the initial chapters and suggest that stress undermines the hormonal system and throws the body out of balance so that PMS can more likely occur. When the individual is stressed, their diet is often out of balance, they tend to eat more sugar, eat more refined foods and baked goods, drink more coffee, more alcohol, and smoke more and indulge in other behaviors that promote PMS.

The goal of a good stress management program should be four fold: 1) reduce stress, 2) eliminate stress wherever possible, 3) educate as to the causes of stress so that stress can be prevented, 4) creation of an active stress-fighting mechanism or set of behaviors so that when under stress the educated individual has number of techniques, or "bag of tricks" to use to reduce, eliminate or prevent coming under the effect of stress. For more information about stress and stress management, go to http://www.PreventiveMedicinePS.com/Stress/.

Lifestyle Intervention

Lifestyle intervention requires that the PMS woman recognizes the many things in her life that she is doing or accepting that are either causing or contributing to her PMS. Above we have talked about a number of these factors, including diet, hormones, stress management, smoking, use of alcohol, relationships, etc. In the broadest possible sense, lifestyle intervention would suggest that we sit down with each PMS woman and look at all of the factors in her life that cause or potentiate her PMS and then one by one, easiest to hardest we create strategies and plans to normalize, control, eliminate and change those factors that are undermining her and contributing to the occurrence and severity of her PMS symptoms.

This is not a usual or commonly available form of treatment performed by most medical doctors. Some psychologist and counselors will work with individuals to provide this type of service.

Surgical Interventions - Removal of the Uterus - Hysterectomy

During the course of discussing treatments of PMS invariably someone will bring up the concept of surgical interventions, specifically total abdominal hysterectomy with or without removal of one or both ovaries. If one looks at statistics for treatment and which treatment gets the best results it is clear that hysterectomy with removal of both ovaries is a major factor is obtaining complete relief from PMS.

It is likely that since PMS is a hormonal problem that removing both ovaries would likely eliminate PMS symptoms most rapidly. There is however, a problem with this logic. Total hysterectomy, as it is called when the uterus and ovaries are removed, is generally not done in women simply to treat PMS. There must be other criteria such as fibroid tumors, endometriosis, irregular bleeding, menstrual pain, uterine polyps, cervical cancer, something that can best be treated by removal of the uterus. Hence improvement of PMS is either a secondary goal or a primary goal with an accepted reason for performing a hysterectomy.

Hysterectomy is a major surgical procedure and while generally quite safe, can be plagued by a list of many complications including death and chronic pelvic pain, therefore should not be done lightly and certainly not for mild or even moderate PMS symptoms.

Removal of a single ovary may or may not help reduce symptoms of PMS, however, once again if removal of an ovary must be done for a complaint other than PMS than reduction of PMS symptoms would be an added benefit.

Removal of the uterus and both ovaries, however, is not an absolute guarantee that all PMS symptoms will be resolved. If the uterus and both ovaries are removed, the PMS woman may immediately be thrown into a surgical menopause with all of the symptoms of menopause potentially occurring. If so, the result may be worse than the original PMS. Lastly, if menopausal symptoms occur this might require starting her on hormone replacement therapy (HRT), and HRT can once again can trigger PMS symptoms as generally synthetic estrogen will likely be used and hence PMS-like symptoms may be triggered in some women.

Anti-Inflammatory Medications

Anti-inflammatory (NSAID's) medications, because they are also prostaglandin inhibitors, do demonstrate relief of some PMS symptoms. When started 3 to 5 days before the onset of PMS, some PMS symptoms are decreased. Medications such as Naprosyn, Motrin, Anaprox, Ponstel, do appear to reduce dysmenorrhea (menstrual cramping) as well. They may, however, be associated with substantial side effects, including stomach upset, indigestion, nausea, vomiting and even gastrointestinal bleeding. It is our belief that they should be used only when no other treatment program works, or when women are unwilling or unable to utilize a dietary approach or more appropriately when NSAID's are indicated for another reason.

A NUTRITIONAL-DIETARY APPROACH TO TREATING PMS

General Dietary Measures

In earlier discussion we have clearly stated that we believe that PMS is a nutritional deficiency-excess syndrome. That is, too little of some nutrients specifically magnesium and vitamin B6 and too much other nutrients such as refined sugars and calcium, in the diet. This however is much too simplistic to tell everything that needs to be told about PMS. Since our nutritional approach is discussed throughout *30-Days to No More PMS* we will not go further in this particular section. In Chapter 5 we will discuss this topic in much greater detail.

The Refined Food Diet and Its Consequences for PMS

A 1983 report found that women with PMS consumed nearly 275% more refined sugar, 79% more dairy products, 78% more sodium, 62% more refined carbohydrates, 77% less magnesium, and 53% less iron than women who did not suffer from PMS. These dietary excesses and deficiencies along with what we have already told you should immediately help to explain why PMS women experience PMS symptoms during in the premenstrual period.

Additionally, beyond their high levels of calcium, which interferes with magnesium absorption, dairy products are also generally quite high in sodium which contributes to fluid retention and aldosterone excess. Refined sugars increase the urinary excretion of magnesium further lowering the amount of circulating magnesium needed to breakdown estrogen into its water soluble conjugated form, potentiating an imbalance between estrogen and progesterone. A heavy intake of sugar also further increases sodium and water retention due to the rapid release of insulin. Dietary salt may exacerbate swelling.

Although conflicting data exist with regard to caffeine and premenstrual breast tenderness, many women find relief if they eliminate or reduce their consumption of caffeinated beverages and foods two weeks before their onset of menstruation. The consumption of caffeine containing beverages is also associated with increases in both the likelihood and severity of PMS among college students. In a study of Chinese women caffeine, due to increased green and black tea consumption, was linked to an increased risk for PMS. Some practitioners recommend a reduction of all caffeine-containing products for women suffering from premenstrual symptoms.

Dietary Fat and PMS

Fiber-rich, low-fat diets are generally most beneficial for women with PMS. They act to reduce the levels of circulating estrogens. As we explained earlier, estrogen is conjugated (turned into its water soluble form) in the liver. Some of it then passes into the small intestine to be elimination in the feces while the rest is collected by the kidney and excreted in the urine. However, bacteria in the intestine reverse the conjugation process remaking estrogen and allowing it to be reabsorbed into the body, back into the blood stream. Fiber-rich, low-fat diets suppress the ability of these intestinal bacteria to do this, ending up increasing the total amount of estrogen excreted in the feces. To date a number of studies have demonstrated that if fat in the diet can be reduced to less than 20% of the total daily caloric intake, this along with increasing fiber in the diet can rapidly reduce blood estrogen levels. A diet high in fruits, vegetables, and whole grains (which also contain lots of magnesium) and low in saturated fat (which caused hardening of the arteries) is a perfect diet for woman with PMS.

More About Magnesium

We have already presented a great deal of evidence regarding the role of a diet high in magnesium in reducing the risk of PMS. We have also told you that women with PMS have been shown to have low levels of magnesium in their red blood cells compared to women who do not suffer from PMS. However, there are few studies that prove, that magnesium alone gives good results. However, the medical world cannot prove this instead they do what we consider to be lack luster empty studies that demonstrate only that they have little understanding of the dietary issues involved in PMS. The following is a good example of what we mean:

> In one randomized, double-blind, placebo-controlled, crossover study (the best type of study according to the medical profession) to evaluate the effect of magnesium on PMS symptoms, a daily supplement of only 200 mg magnesium oxide or a placebo was given to a group of women. Each woman took either the magnesium or the placebo for 2 menstrual cycles (approximately 56 to 60 days). Each patient kept a daily record of her symptoms. The form listed 22 symptoms grouped in 6 groups: 1) PMS-A, 2) PMS-C, 3) PMS-D, 4) PMS-H, 5) PMS-O (other), and 5) PMS-T (total overall symptoms). Urinary magnesium output over a 24-hour period was estimated from spot samples using the magnesium-to-creatinine ratio to assess the patient's overall compliance. No difference was found between the PMS and placebo groups in any symptom category during the first month of supplementation. There was, however, a greater reduction of PMS-H symptoms (weight gain, swelling of the extremities, breast tenderness, abdominal bloating) in the treatment group during the second month compared to placebos.

This is a typical example of planned failure. The amount of magnesium needed to make a difference with PMS when there are no other dietary modifications, where the patient is allowed to continue on their usual refined and processed food diet generally requires 750 mg to 1,000 mg of magnesium daily in order to see results within 30 to 60 days. In this study patient were given only 200 mg of the magnesium, and magnesium oxide which is one of the least well absorbed types of magnesium available in health food stores or markets.

Secondly, since it was not stated that patients were asked to make any dietary modifications we can only assume that they were left to continue hopelessly on their poor, refined and processed food diets. There is no indication as to whether vitamin B6 was added to the diet nor the level of calcium in the diet, nor in fact any other essential vitamins or minerals, nor whether any of these women used birth control pills or have had a tubal ligation, nor how many pregnancies, nor their lifestyles.

In short, this study was a waste of money and time, unless your goal was to publish an article undermining the value of magnesium in treating PMS. Many doctors have very little understanding or knowledge of the role of our daily diets and of magnesium in preventing or reversing PMS. One would like to believe that the people who conducted this study had some knowledge or PMS, diet, the role of calcium and magnesium, but it appears we would be wrong as it is hard to believe any of the people involved in this study had the slightest idea of what they were doing. It is possible that they had another goal in mind as they conducted this study, to prove that medications rather then diet should be used to treat PMS?

Calcium

There are a number of researchers who believe that PMS is caused by a deficiency of calcium in the woman's body. They believe that calcium should be part of the treatment program for all patients with PMS.

It has been our experience that a diet high in calcium will generally worsen the anxiety component of PMS. Some good studies have been done that suggest that overall use of calcium in large amounts can help some women but may worsen PMS symptoms in other women. Instead of a blanket statement that all PMS women should have a diet high in calcium, we suggest instead that a basic diet high in magnesium and relatively high in calcium, that is no more than a total of calcium (between foods and supplements) of 1,200 mg to 1,5000 mg per day (1,299 mg is the calcium equivalent of drinking four glasses of milk each day, along with a health diet), if symptoms improve and there are no problems with any symptoms within two, maximum three months, then great, taking calcium is perfect for you. **Note:** As it takes at least two months of continuous use of calcium before positive or negative results are fully manifested. If anxiety, irritability mood swings or other symptoms of the PMS-A group worsen, then lower the total calcium until either your symptoms go away or your stop using calcium completely. You can get all of the calcium you need from your diet if you know the exact right foods to pick, see our lists of high calcium foods in our dietary section (Table 8). We will discuss how to reduce calcium in your diet in greater detail in the dietary section.

Please also remember, that a diet high in calcium and high in saturated fat can increase your risk of coronary artery disease significantly. This is especially true regarding perimenopausal women with PMS, as quite often their daily diets are low in magnesium and because they are worried about osteoporosis, they are also either taking large amounts of calcium supplements or they are eating large amounts of dairy and dairy products to further increase their calcium intake trying to protect themselves against osteoporosis.

While not entirely pertinent here, it might be helpful for women in their late 40's to know that magnesium forces calcium into the bones, therefore a high calcium diet without magnesium can actually be much less effective in protecting against osteoporosis when compared to a moderate calcium intake (diet and supplements) with 750 mg to 1,000 mg of magnesium daily. This will go a lot further in protecting you from osteoporosis.

One important piece of vital information before moving on. Studies now suggest that woman are much better off obtaining their daily calcium from what they eat and not from supplements. Women who take high levels of calcium supplementation seem to be at considerably greater risk for heart attacks and stroke then women who take in the same amount of calcium but only from their diet. Only use calcium supplements, if you cannot eat sufficient calcium to protect yourself from osteoporosis.

Vitamin B6

Vitamin B6 or pyridoxine is a water-soluble B vitamin which is involved in more than 100 different chemical reactions on a daily basis in your body. Many of these chemical reactions are related to the breakdown, building or metabolism of amino acids and proteins. It is believed that vitamin B6 reduces or eliminates certain PMS symptoms because of its ability to increase the production of serotonin, dopamine and norepinephrine as well as histamine and taurine. Serotonin is important for the regulation of sleep, appetite, and depression. Lowered levels of serotonin and dopamine may play a role in premenstrual symptoms. The use of vitamin B6 in relieving PMS symptoms has been studied extensively. While these studies have suggested that as little as 50 mg a day of vitamin B6 can help many of the symptoms of PMS, especially breast tenderness and breast pain and depression, other studies recommend for best results to use dosages of at least 100 mg per day. An excessive intake of vitamin B6, that is more than 200 mg per day, can cause injury to the small nerves of the legs and hands, that is peripheral neuropathy.

Vitamin E

The specific value of Vitamin E that is helpful in PMS has long been in dispute. Since Vitamin E is present in almost all of the foods recommended in our dietary approach, the point is moot. A number of scientific studies indicate that Vitamin E has no specific value in relieving PMS symptoms when used without other dietary measures. When moderate levels of vitamin E are included about 400 IU, (which happens naturally in our diet plan), vitamin E, which is an antioxidant with other health benefits and minimal side effects, helps to increase oxidation of all foods and improve their utilization by our body. It is safe and can be taken by diet or in supplement form.

Cis-Linoleic Acid

Cis-Linoleic Acid is essential to affect the proper metabolism of sugars, control insulin production and minimize the nervous system's response to any episode of low blood sugar (hypoglycemia). Some people who treat PMS recommend adding foods high in cis-Linoleic acid to the anti-PMS diet. This is a good idea but must be associated with a complete dietary program. On its own, it is insufficient to solve the PMS problem and it can cause a further imbalance if not supported by a balanced and harmonious diet.

OTHER NON-TRADITIONAL MEDICAL APPROACHES

Physical Exercise

Exercise programs generally do not fit well into the medical model of double-blinded, placebo-controlled studies. There have however, been a few studies conducted regarding exercise and PMS, these studies have clearly demonstrated that women who utilize a regular physical exercise program have fewer symptoms of PMS than do women who do not exercise at all. Women who do exercise regularly appear to have improvement in all of the more common symptoms of PMS. These studies have also demonstrated that it is the frequency, rather than the intensity, of the exercise program that appears to bring a meaningful improvement in negative moods and other physical symptoms which may occur during the week to two weeks prior to the onset of menstruation. It is presumed that exercise acts to reduce symptoms by decreasing estrogen levels, decreasing circulating catecholamines (particularly stress hormones), improving blood sugar tolerance, insulin response, and increasing endorphin levels. Once again you can see how changes created by exercise can tie-in directly to a good anti-PMS dietary program. We have created an entire chapter on the role of exercise in the treatment of PMS. See Chapter 7.

HERBAL AND BOTANICAL MEDICATIONS

Before we get to the role of herbs and herbal medicine in the treatment of PMS, we feel that it is important to say a few words about herbal medicines. When we talk about herbs, we have two reference points, first, herbs we eat in our daily diet such as pepper, chilies, cilantro, mint, rosemary, thyme, etc. These are usually eaten in small amounts, known to be edible and safe in the customary amounts in which they are usually used.

The second group is herbal medications. While this group may or may not include some of the edible herbs these are generally considered meaningful because of their medicinal value not their taste or how they change food. Herbal medications are medications, they are in effect drugs all of which must be considered quite potent and potentially dangerous. While we talk about them here as herbs, we also ask you to consider them medications and just like prescription medications should be prescribed and compounded by an expert who knows exactly what he or she is doing, why they are doing it, what the effect of what they are prescribing is going to be, its interrelationships to other medications (both herbal, prescription and over-the-counter) you are taking and its long and short term affects on you. Simply taking herbs from a bottle some health food sales person tells you might or will work for you is dangerous at best and potentially lethal at worst.

Therefore as we discuss herbs we wish to make sure that, as with discussing prescription medications, we are neither suggesting nor prescribing, only educating. If you chose to take an herbal form of treatment for your PMS, good, but be sure it is prescribed, directed and compounded by experts who know exactly what they are doing. Improper use and prescription of herbs can be dangerous. Do not take any chances.

While many herbs are touted as having value in PMS we will concentrate only on the few that have some scientific evidence demonstrating value.

Chastetree (Vitex agnus-castus)

This is an herb which has been used for a long time to relieve menstrual disorders of all types. When tested for its use with PMS, it tested well demonstrating 90% response rate (this includes 33% of PMS women with complete relief of PMS symptoms and 57% with only partial relief). It has been recommended for treatment of depression, breast tenderness, mood swings, food cravings, acne and constipation. There are a limited number of adverse reactions including malaise, gastrointestinal complaints including nausea (most common side effect) and diarrhea.

It is believed that Chastetree works by increasing the levels of LH (luteinizing hormone) which normalizes the second part of the menstrual cycle, restoring progesterone levels to normal and decreasing prolactin levels, hence blocking PMS symptoms. Because of its prolactin inhibiting effect, Chastree may especially be helpful with breast tenderness.

Oil of Evening Primrose

Promoters of Oil of Evening Primrose claim it has great value in eliminating PMS symptoms. It is believed that some of the symptoms of PMS are caused by impaired conversion of linoleic acid into gamma linoleic acid. The goal of using Oil of Primrose is to provide additional essential fatty acids which are safe to support this process. While some women did obtain some relief, there was no scientific study that demonstrated that there was any efficacy in using Oil of Primrose above its placebo effect. We have no objection if any woman wishes to use this substance. However, we usually suggest she save her money and give the dietary approach a try first.

Black Cohosh (Cimicifuga racemosa)

Black cohosh has for years been recommended for the treatment of various symptoms, unrelated to PMS, but some of which do appear to occur in PMS. Of the symptoms which do occur as part of PMS, for example, restlessness, anxiety, tension, nervous excitement, breast pain, menstrual pain and headaches, and depression, black cohosh might well help. Black cohosh has been used for treatment of the symptoms of menopause. Certain varieties of this herb have been shown to act as a mild serotonin reuptake inhibitor hence the reason for its effect in treating depression.

Unfortunately, other recent studies are now suggesting that black cohosh may potentiate some forms of cancer, so at least for the moment the use of black cohosh for any reason is in doubt and it should not be used.

Ginkgo (Ginkgo biloba)

A trial of ginkgo may be attempted if you are experiencing primarily PMS-H, symptoms during your premenstrual period, that is fluid retention, breast tenderness, weight gain. It may prove beneficial as at least one study has suggested statistically significant improvement for the above symptoms. The dosage recommended was 80 mg twice daily from day 16 of the menstrual cycle through day 5 after the menstrual period. Breast tenderness and pain and fluid retention was most benefitted.

St. John's Wort (Hypericum perforatum)

St. John's Wort has been recommended specifically for treatment of depression and irritability during the premenstrual period. When studied St. John's Wart proved to be superior to placebos and as effective as prescription medication for the treatment of mild to moderate depression. When used to treat PMS more than 2/3 of the PMS women using it noted at least 50% decrease in symptoms. The amount of St. John's Wort used in this study was 300 mg three times daily. Adverse reactions to St. John's Wort can include photosensitivity reactions in patients who go out into direct sun light while using this herb.

Kava (Piper methysticum)

Kava is an herb that has been used as a beverage and medicinal agent in the South Pacific for hundreds of years. There have been at least nine clinical studies conducted looking at the use of kava for the relief of anxiety and menopausal irritability. The results have demonstrated that kava has the ability to reduce at least mild anxiety and irritability, symptoms of stress, and restlessness. Kava is found in a number of over-the-counter herbal products sold in the United States for PMS, unfortunately, however there have been no good studies which have looked at kava as a therapeutic agent for PMS, therefore, while it is used in products to treat PMS there is no scientific proof that it actually works. The dose recommended in clinical trials was 100 mg to 200 mg up to 3 times per day.

Other Botanicals Which Are Used to Treat Symptoms Common to PMS

Many different herbs are used in hundreds of preparations which tout themselves as a treatment for PMS complaints. These component herbs may include valerian root, dandelion, Devil's club, blue cohosh (Caulophyllum thalictroides), wild yam (Dioscorea villosa), black haw (Viburnum prunifolium), and pulsatilla (Anemone pulsatilla) and all have for one or another reason for being used to treat many different types of female problems. Unfortunately there is little scientific evidence as to the efficacy of any of these herbs therefore we can neither recommend them nor tell you that they do not work. If you chose to try them, then remember the old saying, "Let the buyer beware."

TREATING PMS WITH ACUPUNCTURE

Of the many non-western medical therapeutic programs for treating PMS the only one which has shown excellent results is acupuncture. The success rate of acupuncture in treating PMS symptoms runs between 60% and 80% depending upon which study you read. The positive influence of acupuncture in treating PMS symptoms is believed to be due to its effects on increasing serotonin and endorphin production and their transmission and increased function throughout the body. The positive results with treating PMS symptoms with this holistic approach are quite encouraging and acupuncture along with a whole food diet combine to provide an excellent and yet entirely safe, method of treatment.

Acupressure and Body-Energy Work

The goal of acupressure is to press upon trigger areas throughout the body. The pressure applied to these trigger areas will either act to release blocked energy, trigger the release of certain neurochemicals, or alter in some way the impaired physiology of the PMS woman. Acupressure can be learned quickly and while best results may be attained when performed by and skilled operators, can be learned and used by the woman herself in the privacy of her own home or wherever she is when she needs it. Once again there are no clearly well done studies that prove its efficacy (ability to work), however given that it is generally considered safe, easy to use and its cost is generally minimal. When you do this along with a good anti-PMS diet, how can you go wrong?

Body-energy work is as old as human beings are, like acupressure it releases energy blocks reduces tension and relieves stress. If you like massage, you will probably like body-energy work. Beware, however, that there are many different schools of body-energy work and massage, some of these schools believe that energy is only released through pain and deep massage, while other schools believe more in a basic pleasure principle and cause little pain and give more of a relaxing and restful massage to release tension. Check with the therapist you will be working with as to his or her beliefs *before* you start and make sure you agree with them.

Both acupressure and body-energy work should be used with a balanced program of diet, exercise for best results in relieving PMS.

DOING NOTHING

The question often comes up, "What if I do nothing? Will my PMS just get better on its own?" There are really two good answers to these questions. The first answer is, if you do nothing you may get better on your own or you may not. The second is, if PMS is any kind of indication of a nutritional deficiency-excess syndrome and there are other consequences, why continue to suffer and run the risk of problems later on. On a practical basis most women with PMS who do nothing generally seem to worsen until late in their 40's then their symptoms change to those of menopause. A woman with difficult PMS symptoms is more likely to also have difficult menopause symptoms. Some people believe that PMS and menopause symptoms are really one condition with two manifestation.

We have throughout the course of this book listed the underlying results of eating a diet which is primarily made up of refined and processed foods, the ultimate physiologic and chemical changes this creates in the body, the consequences of magnesium deficiency, vitamin B6 deficiency and excess of calcium and salt along with the refined food diet. So we will not go deeper into the issue of the second answer. However, there is information from a study done to evaluate the role of placebo's in treating PMS.

PLACEBO STUDIES

A placebo is defined as a medicine prescribed for the psychological benefit of the patient rather than for any physiological effect. In a sense the power of any placebo lies *within the patient's belief in the power or ability of the pill, potion or treatment given to heal them.* It is also a substance that has no therapeutic effect, when used as a control in testing new drugs. When medical research is done, it is generally structured to see how a specific medication works and usually half of the patient in the study are given real, hopefully active, medication while the other half of the patients are given placebos', in the form of an inactive or inert substance. The idea is to find the real effect of the medication verses the "psychological benefit" of taking the pill or whatever form the medication is in.

The goal is to prove that the "real" medication really works and that any side effects that occur from it are also real and not based on any psychological effect. First of all, these type of studies rarely if ever take into consideration that each person is an individual, each has different beliefs, values, levels of pain response and often very different physiologies. Secondly, diet, lifestyle and personal habits are also rarely, if ever, considered in any of these studies.

The study we are about to discuss was looking not at the results of a "real" drug on PMS but rather what would happen to the group of women who only took a placebo. This is a turn on the regular order used routinely in medical research. The results while interesting were not terribly meaningful as the diet, and lifestyle of the individuals taking placebos was not included in what was looked at so we do not who, if any, of the women changed their diet or lifestyle during the course of this project. For what it is worth, here goes:

When a group of women were treated with placebos, 20% of the placebo-treated women showed confirmed improvement in their PMS symptoms. Eighteen of these women took at least 3 of the 4 months of placebo medication before becoming symptom free. Forty-two percent of the women experienced partial improvement, and 39% of this group showed no improved throughout the study period.

Clearly some women who initially demonstrated severe PMS symptoms experienced significant and sustained improvement using only placebo medication, but the majority of the women in this study reported only partial or no improvement. Women who had sustained improvement for a minimum of 2 consecutive months were likely to remain improved, indicating the importance of non-drug factors in the clinical evaluation and treatment of the woman with PMS symptoms.

The researchers conclusion was as follows: "If these same women who showed relief of their symptoms with placebos alone had been subjected to other medical treatment, this would in the end would have subjected them to unneeded risk and danger."

While this study is interesting, it really only tells us one thing in regard to patients who want as little as possible in the way of medical treatment: A trial of dietary treatment for all women would have eliminated or demonstrated significant improvement in these women with PMS symptoms and would have presented no apparent risks nor potential of harm, while at the same time it would have helped them prevent other nutritionally-related medical risks and problems.

A COMBINED APPROACH, ELEMENTS OF TWO OR MORE METHODS LISTED ABOVE

As happens commonly with medical treatment regimes, especially when the underlying cause of the problem is not specifically treated and eliminated, treatment of a medical condition may require multiple approaches and use of more than one medication or modalities of treatment. This is a common problem with PMS.

While we have no difficulty with the use of medications, when they are needed. And, we are aware, as we have stated earlier, that some women would rather be treated through the medical system. We have however, over the years had many experiences with women who have dropped out of our program because they did not wish to give up certain foods, didn't want to change their diet, or because they believed that they had to be treated with medications and through the medical system only. One of these women, was a patient by the name of Janet.

CASE HISTORY #3

Janet was in her late 20's. She had moderately severe PMS with mood swings, anxiety, depression, swelling and breast tenderness each month. She had noticed that her symptoms had gotten worse about two years earlier, after she had her first child. She had breast-fed her daughter for eight months and shortly after she weaned her Janet noticed that her PMS had come back worse than she had ever remembered it.

Janet came in with her husband who had seen us on a television interview program. He was very upset with her episodes of severe anxiety and depression, recognizing that they generally got worse in the week to two weeks before her period, he believed that she might have PMS. After our initial intake we spent a long time discussing the importance of diet, increasing the amount of magnesium and vitamin B6 in the foods she chose to eat and their role in eliminating PMS. Janet listened to everything we said, but appeared distant and unmoved. Later she told us that she was fearful that without a medication, a pill or some kind, she would get no results, however she ultimately agreed that she had to do something about her symptoms. Janet started on our dietary program and within two months the great majority of her PMS symptoms were gone and Janet and her husband were elated.

A month later Janet went to her regular OB/Gyn for her semi-annual checkup. When she told her doctor about the PMS program she was on and how good she was feeling, he told her that being on a diet was "simply foolishness" and that she "should stop it immediately."

Janet trusted her OB/Gyn and became so confused that she ultimately agreed to stop the dietary program and give up. She called us several months later to report that her symptoms had all returned and her depression was worse than ever. As her doctor had told her she would "soon become calcium deficient and that she would be at risk for osteoporosis" on our diet. She was fearful of resuming the dietary program because when was not sure of the risks of less calcium in her diet. We once again explained that she was in no danger of a calcium deficiency as long as she was eating a high magnesium-vitamin B6 diet and taking the PMS vitamin-mineral supplement.

In spite of her husband's urging and our reassurances, Janet refused to return to the dietary program. We never heard from Janet again. We did, however, discover from her husband, later on that her OB-Gyn had put her on a number of medications including a diuretic, progesterone tablets (probably not natural progesterone) and Xanax for her anxiety. The combination did relieve most of her symptoms and she apparently was happy as her progress "pleased her doctor."

There is no question that PMS symptoms can be reduced and in some cases even eliminated by using medications. However, if as we believe is clear, that PMS is a nutritional deficiency-excess syndrome, how does the use of medications really help the woman if in the end her symptoms are reduced or even eliminated, but the underlying cause of her PMS is left unchecked. We believe that we answer this question in Chapter 4 and throughout the course of this book.

THE IDEAL CLINICAL EVALUATION FOR PMS WOMAN

Before any diagnosis of PMS can be made, it is important that each woman suffering from any symptoms attributable to PMS, have a complete medical evaluation for PMS. The evaluation for

PMS should include a careful and complete medical and family medical history, including information regarding mother, sisters, grandmothers regarding menstruation, pregnancy and PMS. The practitioner should in the course of taking a medical history establish of the exact symptoms, exactly when they occur in relation to the menstrual period, the severity of the symptoms, and a detailed evaluation of the woman's level of stress, her diet, how much and how hard she exercises as well as the types of exercise she performs on a regular basis, other known medical problems, use of prescription medications, herbal or over-the-counter medication, alcohol, illicit drugs and overall lifestyle.

A complete physical and pelvic exam should be performed and laboratory tests done to rule out all other potential causes for her symptoms. Testing for prolactin or an adrenal stress test may be considered if the symptom pattern suggests that they are indicated. It often extremely useful for each woman to record her symptoms on a daily basis for at least two complete menstrual cycles in order to see when her symptoms occur, how debilitating or how much of a problem they are, and how they are related to her menstrual cycle.

It is extremely important to address any other underlying medical conditions that may be masked or thought to be caused by PMS. One report found that nearly 75% of women receiving care for PMS at specialized clinics had another diagnosis that accounted for many of their symptoms. Major depression and other mood disorders are commonly misdiagnosed.

TREATMENT OF PMS RELATED MIGRAINE HEADACHES

The level of treatment of PMS related to migraine headaches often depends on the initial diagnosis that in fact the migraines are directly related to PMS. That is if they occur solely during the week to two weeks before the onset of menstruation (the luteal phase) and are associated with other symptoms of PMS and there is no other apparent cause for the migraines. If the migraines occur other then during the luteal phase then they are not likely PMS related and should be treated as per instructions of your physician. Depending on the severity of your symptoms you can take an active role in the management of your PMS related migraine and use the following these guidelines:

- Eat four to six small meals at regular three to four hour intervals. Each meal should be relatively high in complex carbohydrates but definitely low in simple sugars generally found in refined and processed foods, candies and backed goods. This will help your body to maintain a relatively constant blood sugar level and it will help to avoid energy highs and lows.

- Substantially reduce and eliminate, any and if necessary, all use of caffeine, alcohol, salt, fats, and simple sugars to reduce bloating, fatigue, tension and depression (PMS-H Groups symptoms).

- Take a daily vitamin-mineral supplemental containing B6 (at least 100 mg), B complex, magnesium (300 mg-1000 mg), Vitamin E (400 IU) and vitamin C (1000 mg) at least. This combination will help to reduce symptoms of irritability, fluid retention, joint aches, breast tenderness, anxiety, depression and fatigue. Be sure to check with your doctor before taking any other medications for your PMS related migraine headache.

- Exercise is generally helpful for reducing PMS symptoms as it also reduces stress and tension, acts as a mood elevator, provides a sense of well-being and improves blood circulation by increasing natural production of beta-endorphins. It is recommended, if you have no other contraindications that you begin regular exercise program, exercising at least 20-30 minutes three times weekly. Aerobics, walking, jogging, bicycling and swimming are a few of the suggested ways to exercise. See our chapter on Exercise and PMS.

ARE MOST WOMEN SATISFIED WITH TREATMENT PRESCRIBED TO TREAT THEIR PMS?

In a 1998 study which looked at how long it took the average PMS woman to find medical help, how many physicians they saw prior to getting help, and how many physicians actually recognized that they suffered from PMS and needed help, the following was found.

It took the average woman nearly 5½ years or more before receiving a diagnosis of PMS from a medical doctor. She had to seek help from between 3¾ physicians for her PMS symptoms before she found one that could make the diagnosis for her. She would state that the majority, 71% of physicians she saw were too inadequately informed to make the diagnosis of PMS and treat them, Only a minority, some 23% of these physicians used a symptom chart to help them to confirm a diagnosis of PMS, when they were determining what is going on with them. And only approximately 1 in 4, 26% physicians provided them with any helpful treatment.

The study suggested that nearly 76% of subjects reported that a PMS diagnosis resulted from their own suggestion that they have PMS, with subsequent agreement by the physician.

Eighty-one percent reported that the initial suggestion of PMS came from a non-medical source. The most commonly recommended and used treatments were vitamins, exercise, and diet modification.

The study also suggested that only 35% of these women were very satisfied with their treatment, 48.8% were either somewhat satisfied or satisfied with their treatment program and 15.6% were not very satisfied. Satisfaction was higher if natural progesterone or hysterectomy with removal of both ovaries was included as a treatment, although a high percentage of satisfaction was also seen with several other treatments.

SUMMARY

PMS is a nutritional deficiency-excess syndrome. It is caused by a diet depleted in the B vitamins, especially vitamin B6, and the mineral magnesium. These nutritional deficiencies lead to an inability of the liver to break down estrogen. This causes a rise in estrogen and a relative decrease in progesterone. The symptoms of PMS are a sign of these changes and indicate that a nutritional deficiency is present.

A deficiency of vitamin B6 and magnesium can occur in the form of an absolute deficiency created by a diet which is devoid of or, more likely, simply low in B6 and magnesium. It can also be created by a relative deficiency where the diet is proportionally higher in the group of foods which we will refer to as the "Offender Foods." The offender foods are those foods which create a condition that leaves the woman with insufficient nutrients to properly process her estrogen. The offender foods include simple carbohydrates, refined sugars, foods high in calcium and caffeine-rich foods as well as some food additives, food colorings and dyes.

Treatment of PMS requires a clear understanding of the cause of PMS. When PMS is not recognized as a nutritional deficiency-excess syndrome, treatment is generally directed at relief of symptoms only. However, simply relieving symptoms may not eliminate the real problem: the deficiency of vitamin B6 and magnesium.

When the PMS woman is on the right diet for her, her symptoms will simply seem to disappear, as if by magic. However, it is not magic but rather an appropriate diet.

30 Days To No More PMS

In the next chapter we will present the readers of our 30-Days to No More PMS program with the fundamentals of the PMS nutritional program to eliminate PMS. We will offer the information you will need to establish a diet that will protect you from PMS. We will define which foods potentiate PMS and how you can avoid them. You will learn how you can eat whatever you want and still remain symptom free.

The reader should also be aware of the available options in the form of hormonal and non-hormonal medical treatments for PMS. This information is essential in order for the reader to be able to make an educated choice of the type of treatment program she will want to use.

Remember: Approach the treatment of your PMS symptoms wisely. Choose the medical consultant who most represents your views.

Consider your diet *first* as the major culprit in causing PMS. Read this work again until you have developed your own personal plan for evaluating and approaching your PMS symptoms. If you do not get the results you want right away, do not consider it as failure. You may find success simply by modifying what you are doing and looking at where you are not doing what you need to do.

(This Page Is Purposefully Left Blank For You To Use To Take Notes)

CHAPTER 4

UNDERSTANDING THE NUTRITIONAL APPROACH TO TREATING PMS

In the first chapter of our 30-Days to No More PMS program we stated that PMS is caused by a nutritional deficiency-excess and that when this deficiency-excess are corrected your PMS symptoms will simply disappear. This is entirely true. The anti-PMS diet we are about to present to you provides basically all of the nutrients, vitamins and minerals that are needed for your body to function normally and healthfully. It is possibly as close as one can get to the natural diet of mankind. But it is not just a diet to treat PMS. It has a much broader application because it is, in fact, "A good, healthy diet."

We must caution you, though, that it will only work for you if you use it correctly. In a later section we will describe how to do this. It will be our job to make this diet so appealing (if only in relieving your PMS symptoms) that you won't want to think about eating any other way.

In Chapter 2 we discussed the role of the B vitamins, especially vitamin B6, and magnesium in the metabolism of estrogen. We suggested that if adequate amounts of vitamin B6 and magnesium are not available in the foods you eat that estrogen cannot be broken down and excreted as it should be. When this happens estrogen levels rise and, proportionately, progesterone levels fall. Since each woman's body is accustomed to a specific ratio of estrogen to progesterone, the resulting rise of estrogen changes this ratio and thus the body chemistry. In Chapter 1 we described this process in detail. The body responds to the imbalance of this delicate relationship by creating the symptoms of PMS.

In a sense, PMS symptoms are the consequence of the wrong diet for a particular individual. By adjusting the diet so that it is right for your particular needs, your PMS problem can be solved and your PMS symptoms will go away. When this happens, your body will be supplied with exactly what it needs to function normally. The signs and symptoms of precisely the right diet is good health, your sense of well-being and the cessation of your PMS symptoms.

How does the PMS woman eat the wrong diet? While general concepts of what is and is not a good diet are available for large groups of people, what is right and wrong for an individual is not usually very well defined. We have a vast amount of general information about diet. Very little effort, however, has been made by the medical profession to discover what is normal and appropriate for a specific individual. Also, most medical research looks almost entirely at what is abnormal. Even more astounding is that few medical researchers look at what is correct or normal every day nutrition for women suffering from PMS. My (Allen Lawrence) medical school training in nutrition consisted of approximately 6 to 8 hours of class and reading time. It included learning about such nutritional problems, diseases and syndromes as kwashiorkor, scurvy, pellagra, rickets, pernicious anemia and iron deficiency anemia. We also learned about an assortment of vitamin and mineral deficiencies and excesses.

In middle class America, the majority of the conditions listed above are not commonly found. In recent years, nutritional problems such as coronary artery heart disease, stroke, high blood pressure, high cholesterol, diabetes, obesity, arthritis, ulcer and bowel disease have begun to occupy the time and interest of those few physicians who work with diet. As with PMS, many of these problems are correctable by early prescription of a proper diet. But, unfortunately, few medical doctors are aware of what a proper PMS diet is. Even when they are aware, the fact is that they do not have the time to sit down and discuss diet and nutrition with their patients. Worse than that, the medical system is rarely set up to have a nurse or nutritionist available within the practice to do what the medical doctor hasn't the time to do. And, in most cases, insurance companies will not reimburse for these services when they are done.

While our discussion is limited to PMS, the diet we are about to present can also help protect you, your husband or boyfriend and your children against heart disease, diabetes (depending on the genetic make up of the individual), obesity, most vitamin-mineral deficiency syndromes and many other nutritional problems.

The diet that most Americans, and other people around the world, presently eat predisposes them to PMS as well as other dietary deficiency syndromes. We jokingly refer to it as "The Great American Diet." It is high in calcium, fat, refined carbohydrates, refined sugars and salt. It includes processed, canned, frozen and fast foods which may contain large amounts of food additives, preservatives, food dyes and colorings. It has invaded every home in America and has been or is presently being exported into every country in the world.

This "Great American Diet" is usually grossly deficient in proper human nutrition. Time and time again, animal researchers have shown that when this diet is fed to animals it causes them to suffer reduced vitality and to develop a multitude of illnesses. It shortens their natural life spans and causes them to die a quite unpleasant death.

Previously we suggested that the PMS woman could have either a relative or absolute deficiency of those nutrients necessary to eliminate PMS. Absolute deficiencies are fairly common in our society. It most commonly is seen in women who continuously or frequently starve themselves to control their weight. This happens where women are restricting calories and limiting their intake to a specific food. They may be using "fad diets" such as the Grapefruit Diet, Apple Diet, protein powder diets, etc. It can also happen in women who chronically purge themselves. The act of eating in itself is not enough to guarantee good nutrition. Nutrients must not only get into the digestive system but they must be digested and cross over into the blood stream to be useable. If there are little or no essential nutrients in the foods we eat or if they are purged before they can be fully digested they are of no value.

One of the most common reasons for an absolute deficiency occurs because foods are harvested too early, before they are ripe and have their full complement of vitamins, minerals and other nutrients. Foods which are stored for long periods of time, which are frozen, saturated with chemicals, hauled long distances while being exposed to the elements and repeatedly cooked (canned and processed foods) are often deficient in B vitamins and magnesium. If the woman's diet is heavily made up of these foods, she may end up with an absolute deficiency of these important nutrients.

Another frequent reasons for absolute deficiencies are women who are alcoholics. Often these women would rather drink alcohol than eat. Because they are not eating, they are also not able to get proper nutrition. Even those women who do eat "adequately" may still experience a relative deficiency since alcohol is basically pure sugar.

The most common cause of PMS, in our experience, is the relative deficiency situation. There are three main reasons for this. Foods eaten either compete with, use up or inactivate magnesium and vitamin B6. Therefore, a PMS woman may eat a diet that would, under normal conditions, have sufficient amounts of B6 and magnesium, however since they may also eat other foods which actually compete with, use up or inactivate these healthy nutrients, they as a result, become deficient while eating plenty.

Through the remainder of our 30-Days to No More PMS program we are going to designate those foods which we believe are good for you as the "Desired Foods." Those foods which stimulate or worsen PMS, that is, compete with, use up or reduce available vitamin B6 and magnesium, we will refer to them as "Offender Foods," "Undesirable Foods" or "Foods to Be Avoided." We will discuss both categories throughout the remainder of this chapter and the next.

WHAT ARE THE DESIRED FOODS?

They are any and all foods which have more magnesium than calcium. They are foods which are high in Vitamin B6. Desired foods are those which normalize and stabilize the hormonal system and decrease or eliminate PMS. Generally, these foods are whole grains, legumes (beans), cereals, and fresh vegetables and fruits (see the Desired Foods list in Chapter 4). Generally, as a rule of thumb, the fresher these foods are and the closer they were picked or harvested to their due date, the better and the healthier they are.

WHAT ARE THE OFFENDER FOODS, UNDESIRABLE FOODS OR FOODS TO AVOID?

They are the simple carbohydrates, processed and refined foods, alcohol, foods and beverages which are high in sugar and/or caffeine, foods high in calcium, for example dairy products. Certain vegetables, meats and fruits may fall into this category as well. Foods that are fried or have a heavy fat content, such as fast foods, can also worsen PMS. Topping the list is chocolate, of course, because it is high in sugar, calcium, fat, and caffeine. We also suggest you consider food additives, dyes, colorings and preservatives as Offender Foods.

Many women really do not know what a healthy diet is. They generally think of a healthy diet in terms of what they had been taught in relationship to the four food groups. However, the PMS woman needs a diet that contains the right foods, in the right amounts, to relieve her PMS symptoms.

CASE HISTORY #4

Toni was a very athletic person. She ate what *she* considered to be a good healthy diet. Yet for ten days of every month she suffered with headaches and with swelling of her hands, feet and abdomen. She was referred by a friend who suggested that her symptoms might be due to PMS. We surveyed her diet and discovered that she ate a lot of calcium rich fruits and vegetables. She didn't eat much in the way of grains since she believed they were "fattening."

In the beginning it was extremely difficult to get her to understand that although she did eat a very healthy diet, it was one that created lots of PMS symptoms for her. She had little if any high magnesium foods in her diet.

When we first gave Toni the food lists and discussed the importance of increasing her intake of vitamin B6 and magnesium rich foods, she agreed to try the program for one month. During her next cycle Toni noticed that her weight remained the same but her PMS symptoms had lessened significantly.

Due to her fear of gaining weight, Toni went on and off the anti-PMS diet for several months. Six months later, however, she told us that she was going to stay on her new "good, healthy diet" as she clearly felt better on it. What finally convinced her, however, was that she had not gained weight and her athletic performance and endurance had greatly improved.

DEFINITIONS

In order for you to understand our 30-Days to No More PMS program we must spend a little time defining the terms we are using. We will tell you everything you will need to know about magnesium, vitamin B6, calcium, caffeine, carbohydrates, processed foods and alcohol. We will also tell you how and why the foods you choose can overcome your PMS.

Magnesium

Magnesium is an extremely essential mineral that accounts for about .05 percent of the body's total weight. Nearly 70% of the body's supply of magnesium is located in the bones, together with calcium and phosphorus. The other 30% is found in the soft tissues, muscles and body fluids.

Magnesium, as we stated earlier, is extremely important to the proper metabolism of estrogen. However, it is also involved in a number of other important metabolic processes. Two of the most important of these are the metabolism of simple (sugars) and complex carbohydrates, and the metabolism of amino acids, the building blocks of proteins. Magnesium plays an important role in the way our nerves and muscles work. Magnesium also plays a major role in controlling the acid and alkaline balance of the body which is extremely important to our day-to-day survival.

Although magnesium appears to be widely distributed in foods, it is not very abundant in the "Great American Diet" most commonly eaten by the American people. Moreover the foods that most commonly are a part of the "Great American Diet" are foods which generally have a high proportion of empty calorie junk foods, fried foods and fats. In the end, these foods are not only deficient in magnesium, but they are also essentially devoid of most of the meaningful nutrients that interact positively with magnesium and they are high in nutrients that compete, use up or require magnesium for their metabolism.

The most commonly suggested sources of magnesium are raw, unmilled wheat germ, soybeans, figs, corn, apples, millet, brown and wild rice, oil-rich seeds and nuts. For a greatly expanded list see Desired Foods - High Magnesium Foods in Chapter 4. This list is the basis of the anti-PMS diet.

Leafy green vegetables usually thought to be high in magnesium may not be because of cooking, freezing, early picking, or length of time from their harvest to your table. Even more problematic is the fact that, in many agricultural areas, the soil has become so depleted that it no longer has sufficient magnesium or other minerals to provide a good nutritional source.

Vitamin B6

Vitamin B6 is necessary to process estrogen into its inactive form. It facilitates the functioning of linoleic acid in the synthesis of specific prostaglandins associated with estrogen metabolism. Intrinsically connected with vitamin B12 absorption and the production of hydrochloric acid, B6 is critical to the digestive process. B6 is also essential to the body's ability to utilize magnesium. Finally, B6 is also critical to the metabolism of table sugar and other simple carbohydrates which ultimately must be used to provide energy for the brain, liver and muscular tissues especially when the diet is deficient in natural complex sugars. The role of vitamin B6 in the metabolism of blood sugar is essential to the normal function of the body. B6 and magnesium work together to maintain many critical systems, when they are deficient, used up, competed with or inactivated the end result are the problems we call PMS.

Calcium

Calcium is the most abundant mineral in the human body. About 99% is deposited within the bones and teeth. The remaining 1% can be found in the soft tissues, cells and fluids of the body. If it is to function properly, calcium must be accompanied by appropriate amounts of magnesium, phosphorus, and Vitamins A, C, and D. Calcium and magnesium are partners in maintaining cardiovascular and bone health. Calcium is important in the blood clotting process and in muscle growth, muscle contraction, nerve function and impulse transmission. It also plays a role in iron metabolism, while helping to activate several enzymes and regulate the passage of nutrients in and out of the cell wall.

The most abundant sources of calcium are dairy and milk products. However, it is also commonly found in many vegetables and other foods (See Foods to Avoid list, in Chapter 4).

Calcium absorption is generally very inefficient. Only about 20% to 30% of the calcium consumed is absorbed. Milk, once thought to be an excellent source of calcium, is now known to be a poor source of available calcium because of its high levels of potassium and phosphorus.

Even with its difficulty in being absorbed calcium is approximately ten times more abundant than magnesium in the average diet and 15 to 20 times more common in the foods that make up the usual diet of women with PMS. The key to a good anti-PMS diet is in the ingestion of at least two units of magnesium to every unit of calcium in order to eliminate or to prevent PMS symptoms. It may now be easier to see why it is so important to reduce dietary calcium and increase dietary magnesium. The diet we suggest is not a low calcium diet, but rather a diet with a better balance between calcium and magnesium.

Another well-known fact is that calcium and magnesium are antagonistic to each other. As the blood levels of calcium rise, magnesium is pushed into tissues making it unavailable for biochemical reaction. As magnesium levels rise, calcium is pushed into the bone where it is stored and used to make the woman's bones stronger.

If the diet is poor in magnesium, calcium may actually be pulled out of bone tissue thereby weakening the bones. When the diet is too high in calcium, the excess in the bloodstream can compete with magnesium for certain binding sites. The metabolic process in action can then be blocked, stopped or routed in a new direction. It is as if magnesium is unavailable even when magnesium is plentiful in the system. Calcium specifically pushes magnesium away from the sites where magnesium must bind if it is to protect the woman from PMS.

Carbohydrates

Carbohydrates are made up of three types of substances: cellulose, sugars and starches. Cellulose, also known as fiber, is essential to proper functioning of the intestinal tract, to the formation of stool and to the prevention of bowel diseases and bowel cancer. While most types of fiber are not digestible, some types are and they affect the body's level of cholesterol. The main effect of fiber on PMS is its role in clearing estrogen from the blood when on a diet high in fiber, 25 to 30 grams per day, women usually experience a reduction in or a complete end to their PMS symptoms. Interestingly enough, most high magnesium foods have a high fiber content.

Another area which is vital to the PMS woman is sugar. This is a general name for a group of carbohydrates. There are simple sugars and complex sugars. Simple sugars are also more difficult to break down and digest while complex sugars are easier and more naturally digested by the human body. Simple sugars are any sugar that has been processed in any way. Complex sugars are usually natural sugars found in unaltered fruits and vegetables.

Refined Sugar and Starches

We are most concerned with the two groups of carbohydrates, the complex and refined carbohydrates. We can further break down each of these two groups into complex sugars, fibers and starches, and refined sugars and starches. The complex carbohydrates are all natural unadulterated carbohydrates, for example: vegetables, fruits, potatoes, corn and so on. The refined or processed carbohydrates include all other carbohydrates, those that have in anyway been altered by any commercial process, cooking, food processing or manufacturing. Within the refined carbohydrate groups we are specifically interested in the refined sugars, specifically foods like table sugar, white and brown sugar, turbinado sugar, molasses, honey, white flour, polished white rice (see the list in Table 5) and the foods and products that contain them: candy (especially chocolate), cookies, cakes and pastries, regular non-diet soda drinks, alcohol, jams, jellies, syrups (even syrups in medicines), and all of the hundreds of other foods that contain refined sugars and starches.

These refined or processed sugars and starches are also commonly referred to as simple carbohydrates. The term simply refers to the changes in their molecular structure which breaks the natural chains of carbohydrates, referred to as complex carbohydrates, into smaller, more simple groups. Simple carbohydrates are actually more difficult to digest and less natural to the body.

While the distinction between simple and complex may seem small, it makes an extreme difference to the body. The body actually works harder in trying to break down simple carbohydrates. Another distinction is that during the processing procedure, complex carbohydrates are artificially broken down. In these processed foods, the chemicals, heat and pressures that are used often destroy the vitamins and minerals inherent in the parent foods. The process of milling white flour removes the hull, the germ, and the bran of the grain, this along with the bleaching process removes and literally destroys all of its magnesium and vitamin B6.

For future reference when we refer to sugar, we are referring to **ALL** foods that act like a 'sugar' (simple carbohydrate) when the body metabolizes them. We, however, include some foods which you might not have previously considered to be a sugar, such as white rice and white flour. This concept is often difficult to get accustomed to. However, to assure the best possible results in treating PMS, you will need to think differently. If you are going to eliminate those foods that promote PMS from your diet, you must know what they are and why they are a problem.

For our purposes we must now consider that all of the processed foods listed above, as well as any foods which may end in -ose: maltose, sucrose, and dextrose, to be treated as simple sugars. Often, when the so-called natural sugar, i.e., fructose, is added to foods which are either processed or completely artificial, it too should be considered a simple sugar. When natural foods such as carrots, beets, honey, or fruits are cooked and stored for long periods of time or packed under great pressure, these "natural sugars" should be considered simple sugars.

Here's another general rule, foods in a package or a can, mixed with artificial ingredients, cooked or recombined, or foods that require you to add something, including water should be considered processed or refined foods. These foods should be strictly avoided during the second part of the cycle by all women with mild PMS, and avoided all month by women with severe PMS.

Processed and refined foods tend to act like simple carbohydrates. Their treatment in processing and refining tends to change their complex carbohydrates into simple carbohydrates. This, along with the fact that cooking and processing often rob them of much, if not all, of their vitamins and minerals, makes them especially dangerous for the PMS woman.

It should now be very obvious that the PMS woman should learn how to read labels and look for ingredients such as: sugar, honey, corn sweetener, corn syrup, molasses, fructose, dextrose, maltose, dextro-maltose, barley sweetener, modified corn starch, modified food starch, white flour, bleached flour, white rice, rice flour, rice vinegar and rice sweetener. These are all simple carbohydrates, i.e., sugars. (See Table 5, below.)

Sugar Found in Foods in the Following Forms

White table sugar, turbinado sugar, brown sugar, honey, molasses, corn sweetener, corn syrup, any foods which may end in -ose: fructose, dextrose, maltose, dextro-maltose or malto-dextrose, barley sweetener, corn starch and modified food starches, alcohol, white flour, bleached flour, white rice, rice flour, rice vinegar and rice sweetener and processed mashed potatoes.

Table 5

Symptoms such as cravings for sweets and hypoglycemia (low blood sugar) with fainting, sweating, dizziness, palpitations, or headaches should suggest excessive refined sugar intake.

The foods we eat, especially the simple and complex carbohydrates, are first broken down and *digested* by the stomach. The digested carbohydrates go directly to the liver where they are changed into a substance called glycogen. Glycogen is stored in the liver and eventually transformed into glucose or *blood sugar*. The brain can only use glucose as its source of energy. Unlike natural sugars and complex carbohydrates, refined (simple) sugars require a complicated process to be transformed into glycogen. This series of processes requires magnesium and vitamin B6 in addition to many other nutrients. To generate the same amount of blood sugar, the digestion and transformation of simple carbohydrates require more vitamins and minerals and is ultimately much more taxing on the body.

It should now be apparent why the need for vitamin B6 and magnesium becomes greater as the diet increases in refined and processed foods. Any breakdown in the mechanism controlling glycogen may cause sudden fluctuations in blood sugar. These fluctuations can act as a signal of an increased need for energy. This is translated by the body into a craving for sweets. When the PMS woman responds to these cravings by eating more refined sugars, she will also create the release of insulin to manage her blood sugar levels. Therefore more refined sugar she eats, the greater the amount of insulin needed. As insulin pours out circulating sugars are immediately burned up and the process repeats itself again and again until a normal blood sugar is reestablished. This specific faulty pattern accounts for the profound persistent cravings which often occur in PMS.

Often food manufacturers will try to fool the general public. For example, they may sell breads made with 90% to 95% of white, bleached flour and 5% to 10% of whole wheat flour as whole wheat bread. However, since so much of the flour in it has been bleached and milled, it will act as a simple carbohydrate and will have an extremely low level of natural vitamins and minerals.

CHOCOLATE

The primary defect in PMS is the imbalance of nutrients, especially the deficiency of magnesium and B6, along with the excess of calcium, refined foods, simple sugars and caffeine in the PMS woman's diet. Chocolate has all of these. Chocolate is high in magnesium, therefore, even a little chocolate can trigger craving for the magnesium within the chocolate. Chocolate is also high in calcium (milk chocolate), refined (or simple) sugars and caffeine. Since magnesium is essential for the metabolism of sugar and when it is deficient sugar cannot be appropriately broken down. Hence for the PMS woman whose diet is generally low in magnesium, chocolate will trigger a craving for the magnesium which is in it. However, the sugar, calcium and caffeine use up this magnesium and more resulting in an increased deficiency of magnesium, thus creating a vicious cycle. The more chocolate you eat the more you will crave it, the more you crave it the more you will accentuate the deficiency that creates PMS, hence the worse your PMS will become. The rest is easy to follow.

Over the years we have found that many women believe that they love chocolate and that they could not possibly live without it. We remember one woman whose opening statement to us was, "I'll do anything to get rid of my PMS, except give up my chocolate." Our answer was, "Great you do not have to give up your chocolate, you can eat all you want."

What she didn't know and we did, was that once she was on the exact right diet for what her body needed she would naturally lose her cravings for chocolate. We started her on a healthy anti-PMS diet, supplements and got her to reduce the total amounts of other offending foods in her diet, within one month she told us, "I haven't the slightest idea what I ever saw in chocolate to begin with."

Actually this is quite common. Once your diet provides adequate magnesium and other essential nutrients, most PMS women just naturally lose their craving for chocolate. This allows them to eat chocolate whenever they want and it is no longer a problem.

FORTIFIED PRODUCTS

The PMS woman should beware of any product which is labeled *"fortified."* That term generally means either that the original high levels of natural nutrients have been removed and lower levels replaced into it, or that the product naturally has a low level of nutrients and some have had to be added to it to pass FDA requirements in order to sell as a certain category of food. In most situations the product ends up with fewer available nutrients than it had when it was in its natural unprocessed state had it even existed in nature to begin with. In order for it to be advertised as a food, its nutritional value must in some way be increased, so vitamins and minerals may have been added to meet the requirements of the law. Usually these vitamin and mineral nutrients which have been added are in a cheap and poorly available form and are almost always in levels well below the Department of Agriculture's, Required Daily Allowances (RDA) amounts.

ALCOHOL AND PMS

Alcohol must be addressed on its own. By alcohol we mean wine, beer, hard liquor, and any fermented beverages (processed spirits or sugars), not to mention their mixers. Not only does alcohol have an action similar to refined sugar, but it also has specific problems of its own.

The biggest problem is based on the fact that PMS women are often quick to find that alcohol can relieve PMS symptoms. Alcohol acts like a sudden infusion of sugar, causing the blood glucose levels to rise. This rise however, does not last for a very long time and may soon drop away. When this happens, another drink is often necessary to recapture the desired effects. Alcohol, however, has addictive qualities. Over the years we have seen a number of women who have become alcoholics while trying only to get some temporary relief from their PMS symptoms.

This mechanism may be responsible for a substantial number of women becoming alcoholics. Alcohol, in itself, is well known to produce deficiencies in magnesium and the B-complex vitamins, as well as other vitamin-mineral deficiency syndromes, thus potentiating the PMS and worsening the whole process.

CAFFEINE

Caffeine worsens PMS in two ways. It stimulates the stress response thereby causing the release of adrenalin and it creates alterations in blood sugar levels. These mechanisms require an increased use of and need for magnesium. Caffeine itself needs B vitamins for its breakdown and metabolism. Therefore, a diet high in caffeine increases the relative deficiencies of magnesium and B vitamins. Another action of caffeine is its tendency to decrease the appetite. This initially leads to reduced eating and possibly starvation. However, as it wears off there may be a *rebound hypoglycemia* (lowering of blood sugar). When blood sugar levels are lowered, the body signals the *appestat* (the appetite control center). This causes increased cravings for sweets and subsequent overeating. Because of this process, a diet high in caffeine often leads to further nutritional imbalances and deficiencies. The result is a worsening of the problems and symptoms of PMS. (See Appendix E.)

A FRAGILE BALANCE

The balance between the foods ingested and the symptoms they provoke can be very fragile. Sometimes a small amount of offending foods can produce a noticeable change in symptoms. In certain circumstance's compromise is necessary to solve a problem. One of our patients, Madeline W., had such a problem, working together we ultimately solved it.

CASE HISTORY #5

We first met Madeline the day after her 27th birthday. The night before, her boyfriend, Mark, had taken her to a very expensive and romantic restaurant. He had planned to take her to a play afterward but, unfortunately, because of a terrible argument they never got there. During dinner, Mark told her that he had planned a fishing trip over the upcoming weekend. Madeline immediately accused him of being unfaithful (which was not true). Mark finally told her that the reason he was going was because he could tell by her moods when her period was due and he didn't want to be around her at that time. She reacted to this by being argumentative, angry and feeling all alone.

Mark also told her that she needed help and it was he who brought her to see us. After evaluating her, we determined that she did indeed have moderately severe PMS.

Madeline's moodiness and irritability during the week before her period often alienated her from her friends and co-workers. As a hotel concierge, she took pride in doing a great job, but when she was in her premenstrual phase she was reckless, had a short fuse and created problems in both her professional and personal life.

Initially Madeline admitted that each day she was drinking six to eight cups of coffee with cream and sugar, and frequently eating candy bars to sustain her through the day. This seemed like a good reason why she was having PMS. We explained how these foods can aggravate PMS. Within a short while she was able to change to decaffeinated coffee and eliminate the cream and sugar.

We also discussed ways that she could eat at the hotel and remain on the anti-PMS diet. She soon learned that she could request the chef to make some special dishes for her. Since Madeline was not a very good cook, nor was she very inventive as she almost always ate out. With our help she found that she could purchase some good foods at a local health food store and easily prepare them when she got home.

Within a short time these dietary changes made a great difference in her job performance. Her boss's next review of her was glowing. Her boyfriend was more available throughout the month and their relationship got more serious. However, she continued to have irritability during her premenstrual phase that she couldn't seem to get rid of.

We then asked Madeline to restart keeping a daily diary of all the foods she ate. When she returned to our office a few weeks later, we discovered that she had a particular craving for sourdough bread (which is made with processed white flour and dairy). This was apparently enough to throw her delicate balance off. Since she refused to give up her sourdough bread, we suggested that she add vitamin-mineral supplements to compensate for it. Within the next thirty days her symptoms were entirely gone. She was so thrilled that she started telling all

88

her friends of her success in conquering PMS.

Hopefully, through this discussion of definitions we have now clearly shown how important a role magnesium, vitamin B6, calcium, simple carbohydrates and caffeine can play in both creating and eliminating the problems and symptoms of PMS. Also, how fragile nutritional systems may be, in some women.

DIET AND THE FOUR TYPES OF PMS

Earlier we introduced the four types of PMS symptoms: PMS - A, *Anxiety Group*, PMS - H, the *Hydrous (the water retention and swelling) Group*, PMS - C, the *Cravings Group* and, finally, PMS - D. the *Depression Group*. In each of these groups the effects of dietary deficiencies or excesses are the driving forces. It is through your symptoms that you will be able to determine exactly what and how much of a particular food you should and shouldn't eat. When your symptoms disappear you will know that you are on the correct diet *for you*.

PMS-A ANXIETY GROUP

The *Anxiety Group* relates both to deficiencies of magnesium and B6 and excesses of simple carbohydrates. These deficiencies are created specifically by high levels of estrogen and a deficiency of progesterone. The symptoms of this group are characterized by feeling "out of control," or the so-called, Dr. Jekyll-Mr. Hyde behavior changes, episodes of anxiety, nervousness and nervous tension, irritability, emotional liability and mood swings. Women who experience these symptoms, starting one day to two weeks prior to menstruation and lasting until shortly after the onset of menstruation, generally have too much estrogen and too little progesterone in their systems. Estrogen is a stimulant to the nervous system producing a stress-like reaction causing increased tension. The stimulation acts as a stressor causing adrenaline to be released. This stress-like reaction can alter blood sugar levels, creating hypoglycemia (low blood sugar), which worsens the whole process.

Progesterone, on the other hand, is a relaxant to the nervous system.

When progesterone levels are read by the body as decreased (that is either because of an actual reduction of progesterone being produced or because of increased levels of estrogen, or an increased estrogen-progesterone ratio) the balance of activity within the woman changes toward increased stimulation of all systems and most especially the nervous system and you have a PMS-A effect. When the progesterone-estrogen levels are altered to create an increase of *progestogenic* effect and a reduction of *estrogenic* effect, that is, progesterone dominates, these same systems slow down and when it reaches a critical level depression is the end result (progesterone levels high, estrogen levels low) and we have a PMS-D effect.

These negative changes can be controlled by reducing simple carbohydrates and eating 4 to 6 small meals each day. These smaller meals, the sum total of what the individual normally eats only divided into smaller portions, can help to control blood sugar levels and reduce the symptoms commonly associated with the anxiety group.

PMS-H THE HYDROUS OR HYDRATION GROUP

The **Hydrous Group** is produced by an increase of an adrenal gland hormones, ACTH and aldosterone. ACTH and aldosterone controls water and salt retention and potassium excretion by the kidney. The end result is water retention. Often women report abdominal bloating, swelling of the hands and feet, weight gain, headaches, migraine headaches, heaviness, and breast tenderness and fullness. The elevated levels of aldosterone are likely caused by excess estrogen and are facilitated by increased salt intake in the diet, especially in refined and processed foods which are already high in salt. Stress and magnesium deficiency are often additional causes. The adrenal gland is the stress gland. An excessive intake of refined carbohydrates also leads to increased insulin secretion. Insulin causes further retention of salt by the kidney. Once again the interrelationship of diet to the physical symptoms of PMS demonstrates the role of diet in its treatment.

PMS-C THE CRAVINGS OR CARBOHYDRATE CRAVING GROUP

The **Cravings Group** is associated with increased appetite and cravings for foods high in sugar, cookies, cakes, and other sweets, particularly chocolate, also cravings for dairy products, for example ice cream, cheese and yogurt. Women in this group may also crave alcohol in place of sweets or dairy or some combination of the three of these with other foods as well. These cravings are directly related to the menstrual cycle and the overall diet. Headaches, loss of energy, fatigue and pounding of the heart are frequently part of the complex of this group. When a woman who manifests these symptoms eats a diet high in sugar, which is usually at times of stress, it changes the levels of certain enzymes within the brain as we have discussed earlier. The responses of these chemical changes set into motion a vicious cycle of stimulation and suppression of multiple hormones throughout the body. This leads to the symptoms associated with this group. While the exact etiology of this group is unclear, it is believed that it is most likely associated with a magnesium deficiency, or a diet high in refined sugars, enhanced intracellular binding of insulin or inefficient insulin activity, hence blood sugar rises and falls and in the woman ends up craving sugar and sweets.

PMS-D THE DEPRESSION GROUP

The *Depression Group* differs from the previous groups in that it is caused by decreased blood levels of estrogen and increased blood levels of progesterone (the increased progestogenic effect was discussed above) and adrenal androgens (male hormones) leading to an increased break down of neurotransmitters, specifically serotonin. Chronic stress is most likely the trigger which causes the production of certain stress hormones which block the production of estrogen. If there is a specific nutritional deficiency associated with this group, it is not yet clearly defined. A good healthy diet, regular exercise, vitamin-mineral supplements and a small amount of estrogen can help a lot. Most important to this group is relief of stress through therapy. Besides depression other common symptoms in this group include: clumsiness, forgetfulness, need to withdraw, feeling fearful, paranoia, suicidal thoughts and on rare occasions, suicidal acting out may both be successfully or merely used as a show or cry for help. Acting out and suicidal behaviors are both more common in teen PMS girls. See the section on teens and adolescent PMS suffers, in Chapter 6, Section II, Social and Spiritual Problems Related to PMS.

HORMONAL VERSUS DIETARY APPROACH

You might at this point ask which approach is better, hormonal or dietary? Both approaches work! However, we believe that the dietary approach is preferred. Progesterone, although widely used, is not yet approved by the FDA for treatment of PMS. It is also more costly and requires self-medication and relatively frequent medical visits. But these are not the main reasons that we suggest the dietary approach.

There is a large body of knowledge, some of which we have tried to share with you above, is now available showing that nutrition is extremely important to the quality of our life and our health. The sole use of natural progesterone does not relieve either the magnesium or vitamin B6 deficiencies, nor does it necessarily diminish the use of excessive sugar, caffeine or calcium in the diet that caused your PMS originally. Magnesium deficiency is now recognized as a leading factor in heart disease. The proper functioning of the cellular membranes and of the digestive, genital, urinary, skin and immunologic systems as well as bone metabolism, pregnancy and the development of the fetus, are dependent upon adequate amounts of magnesium in the body. Magnesium is so extremely important that it is also called the anti-stress mineral. For these reasons, even though natural progesterone works, we would rather see all women use the nutritional approach for good health maintenance and disease prevention.

We have completed most of the preparation that we believe is necessary for you to understand the how, what, and why of the anti-PMS diet. You now know more about PMS and the diet that prevents and eliminates it than most medical doctors know. Now that we have laid the groundwork, the next and most important step is to start on the anti-PMS diet.

PREPARING YOU TO START THE ANTI-PMS DIET

When we initially started working with women who suffered from PMS we used a dietary program which was recommended by a number of other PMS programs (see Table 6). Often quite simple, these programs relied heavily on the use of vitamin-mineral supplements. In addition to using supplements women were told to increase their dietary intake of foods which were high in vitamin B6 (leafy green vegetables) and high in magnesium (whole grains, legumes and cereals). Most programs advised limiting the consumption of refined sugar, dairy products, salt, alcohol, coffee, tea, chocolate, red meats and fats. We continue to see these same dietary instructions in current books about PMS. In fact, these instructions have changed very little over the years.

During the past 20 years, however, our personal experience has taught us that while these general instructions are sound they are not entirely sufficient. In order to obtain complete symptom relief through a dietary approach the individual woman must become fully aware of the foods she eats and how they affect her mind and body. We have found that many foods not usually considered to be sugars, act like sugar. Some examples are white flour, white rice and processed foods we have mentioned earlier. On occasion in some women even fruits, which are normally considered perfectly healthy, may worsen these PMS symptoms.

We have also discovered that many green, leafy vegetables and other foods high in magnesium will also contain significant amounts of calcium. Because of this, they may actually worsen a woman's PMS symptoms. After cooking and processing, we realized, foods high in magnesium and vitamin B6 may become worthless. These factors were often not accounted for and because of this many women did not get the good results they expected from the dietary approach.

Through the years our patients have been our best teachers. As we were presented with problems and questions by our patients we learned, grew and modified our dietary program until it became consistently successful.

We believe that an important part of treating any woman who wants to use our dietary program is the comprehensive information on what PMS is. We feel that women need to know how it affects them, how it is diagnosed and the various treatments used for it. We have included the basics of this program as the substance of our 30-Days to No More PMS program. But even more important is helping them to understand which foods and style of eating worsens or which improves their PMS.

In our program, we closely monitor each woman for six to eight weeks. We answer her questions, helping her solve the necessary problems until she has learned what works for her and how to consistently reproduce it. We help her learn how to modify the program when necessary to suit her own particular needs.

The last step of our program is to teach her how she can cheat. That is, how she can manage temporarily going off the dietary program and still remain symptom free. Most important of all is that we encourage her to consider that the changes she is making are her own choices. The diet and life style changes that are necessary to make the program work, are to be her life.

We have found that it is extremely important that everything you do should be done out of choice and desire and that it all becomes integrated into your life. If you don't do this, you may always resent these changes and feel as if you are being restricted and punished. This can ultimately defeat you and leave you with your PMS symptoms.

A good example of the types of challenges that can arise during the treatment of PMS is brought to mind in the story of Sandi.

GENERAL PMS DIETARY (NUTRITIONAL) GUIDELINES

1. Eat 6 (six) small meals rather than 2 or 3 large meals each day.

2. 60-70% of daily calories should come from complex carbohydrates (grains, legumes and cereals).

3. Use fish, poultry, whole grains and legumes as your major sources of protein. Consume *no more than* 3 oz. of red meats per week.

4. Limit dairy products to *no more than* 2 (two) servings per week (8 oz. milk or 2 oz. cheese = 1 serving).

5. Limit refined sugar to *no more than* 5 tsp. per day. Refined sugar = white sugar, honey, brown sugar, turbinado or raw sugar, molasses, sucrose, lactose, dextrose, maltose, fructose, corn syrup and sweetener.

6. Limit alcohol consumption to *no more than* 1 oz. per week if at all.

7. Do *not* over salt foods. Rather than cooking with salt add to taste afterward.

8. Use corn margarine or safflower oil margarine instead of butter.

9. *Avoid* processed foods or bleached/white flours and grains as they provide empty calories and may be metabolized as simple carbohydrates.

10. Use 1 tbsp. cold pressed safflower oil each day as a source of cis-linoleic acid. This is especially valuable for women who have problem menstrual cramping.

11. Drink *at least* 4-6 (8 oz.) glasses of water each day or more.

12. Most important *eliminate* caffeine rich foods and drinks (coffee, tea, colas and chocolates).

Table 6

CASE HISTORY #6

Sandi was a 25-year-old single woman who suffered with moderate PMS. As a sales representative for a large electronics firm, she was required to travel extensively. Not only was she at the mercy of hotel food but her job required her to attend large conventions and product shows. It was snack bars and vending machines during the day and fancy restaurants, drinking and socializing with the movers and shakers in the evening.

After three years of living this way she began dreading her trips. She recognized that she was paying a dear price for all of the partying as her PMS was steadily worsening and her self-image was deteriorating.

Because of her lifestyle, Sandi turned out to be quite a challenge. However, she was very motivated and we were able to teach her how to choose anti-PMS foods when eating out and entertaining at trade shows.

When Sandi returned from her trips, we could always tell how well it went for her by how her symptoms were for that cycle. It seemed that when she had a particularly good business trip, she had no problem choosing the right foods. But whenever she became depressed about a potential outcome she would be more careless about her diet.

Prior to treatment she had considered a career change which would not require so much travel. Eventually, she discovered that she was really best suited for the career she had chosen and it was only her diet that she had to change.

She also realized that by getting rid of her PMS she was better able to function in her professional capacity and was ultimately more successful in all aspects of her life. When we last saw her, she was fully able to control her symptoms and was essentially symptom-free.

If you were a patient of ours in our counseling program, we would personally review all of the material we have presented to you above. However, we believe that you have demonstrated your interest and motivation by purchasing our 30-Days to No More PMS program and reading it to this point. If you do adopt our dietary program, do it willingly and do it to the best of your ability.

Now that we have given you a broad overview of the dietary program, we will start you on the path of becoming symptom free. You now know that what you eat is important. What you have eaten in the past caused your PMS and what you eat in the future will eliminate it.

> **What You Have Eaten in the Past Caused Your PMS and What You Eat in the Future Will Eliminate It.**

Summary

To summarize, the secret to complete relief of symptoms is understanding that your body requires magnesium and vitamin B6 to metabolize estrogen. Some of these nutrients are supplied by our diet. By increasing the high magnesium and high vitaminB6 foods, by using supplements and by decreasing the competing foods (high calcium foods, processed foods, sugars, other simple carbohydrates, and caffeine-rich foods and beverages), symptoms can be completely eliminated. To insure this there must be sufficient magnesium/B6 available either in the form of foods or food supplements to properly metabolize estrogen and re-establish your normal *estrogen to progesterone ratio*.

We have found that a key factor is also the *ratio of magnesium to calcium* in your diet. This ratio must be at least two magnesium to one calcium at each meal, including snacks. This is extremely important and cannot be overstated as an essential element in obtaining complete relief of PMS symptoms.

There is no magic in relieving PMS symptoms. The use of natural progesterone, diuretics, tranquilizers, and suppression of ovulation can all be extremely valuable. However, while your symptoms may be relieved, any underlying vitamin-mineral deficiency syndrome will not end up being treated unless you change your diet or take relatively large doses of vitamin-mineral supplements.

All of the PMS symptoms listed in Chapter 1 have logical reasons. They are entirely based on biochemical changes caused either by deficiencies of vitamin B6 and magnesium or by excesses of calcium and foods which use up, compete with or inactivate vitamin B6 and magnesium.

Finally, by this time you should also be aware that certain foods which otherwise appear to be perfectly healthful may potentiate your PMS. In the next chapter we will introduce you to three extremely important food lists, Desired Foods, Neutral Foods and Foods To Avoid. We will demonstrate how to use these lists to choose foods that will not only help you to eliminate your PMS but also to eat and feel better than you ever have before.

(This Page Is Purposefully Left Blank For You To Use To Take Notes)

CHAPTER 5

FOODS TO AVOID ... FOODS TO EAT

Up to this point we have discussed the basics of what PMS is and its cause. The next step is to tell you how to eliminate your PMS symptoms and how to put all of the information we have given you to use. Fortunately, the best way to eliminate PMS is by eating all you want of those healthful nutritious foods that provide you with the nutrients you need to reduce or eliminate your hormonal problems. This will certainly eliminate an absolute deficiency, *if* this is your problem. Since it is more likely that your PMS is caused by a relative deficiency, you must also add another step. You must cut out or significantly reduce those foods which potentiate PMS. And those foods, which we call Offender Foods, are the simple carbohydrates, processed foods, excessive dairy products, and foods and beverages with caffeine and alcohol and foods which contain food additives, dyes, colorings and preservatives as we discussed earlier. Most foods and food products in boxes, cans, TV dinners, packed in cellophane, precooked or manufactured are generally processed and refined foods. This may or may not include foods you might eat in a restaurant except when they are pre-prepared, come from a can, a box or cardboard container and made commercially. It may or may not apply to foods you yourself make in your own home, especially if they contain processed and refined foods.

At this point in our counseling process we are always aware that there are four types of women who sit in front of us.

1. Women who will do everything necessary to eliminate their PMS symptoms.
2. Women who will do some of what is necessary to relieve their PMS symptoms.
3. Women who resent the impositions of the diet and make only a half-hearted attempt at it.
4. Women who expect an overnight miracle or quick fix done for them are usually not willing to change their diet nor their lifestyle.

The first group of women are the easiest to work with. They are motivated and they are usually self-loving. They are willing to put forth whatever effort is needed into getting the job done.

The second group is also generally relatively easy to work with. Often they are less trusting of themselves and the dietary process. They may have a slightly lower self-image. Unconsciously, they may believe either that they are not fully worthy nor capable of getting rid of their PMS symptoms, or that they are not going to be able to eliminate their symptoms no matter what they do. However, these women usually do trust themselves and us enough to try.

The third group is more complex in nature. The women in this group we have found generally have a relatively low self-image. Like the second group, they often lack trust in themselves and others around them. However, they are more likely to project it outside of themselves. They may often make statements like, "I like my chocolates and I am not willing to give them up for anybody!" The "anybody" here is presumed to mean "us." We have two standard answers to this kind of statement: 1) "It is perfectly OK with us if you keep your PMS symptoms. We have no interest in taking them away from you. However, if and when you are ready to give them up, we will be more than willing to help you." 2) It is okay with us, but if you really want to eliminate your PMS, you should at least consider doing what we say.

The last group is often the hardest, and yet also the most rewarding of the four groups. They often resist completely changing their diet and giving up certain offender foods. But when they finally do give the program a try, they usually demonstrate the most dramatic results and are the most appreciative.

Sometimes resistance comes from fearing change and giving up the foods that we are accustomed to. Other times, resistance can come from outside of us, family members or friends. The story of one of our resistant patients, Jennifer, provides a picture of what can happen when this occurs.

CASE HISTORY #7

Jennifer was a 35-year-old grade school teacher who suffered from severe PMS for ten to twelve days each month before her period. During this time she had difficulty controlling her temper, her skin would break out, she craved chocolate and other sweets and, always hungry, she felt like she was a vampire and was constantly eating. Because of her poor eating habits, she would gain weight, become bloated and feel miserable about herself. Eventually her personality changed so drastically that her husband, children and students complained, which simply triggered more anger during her PMS phase and deep humiliation and frustration once her period finally came.

Jennifer was at her wits' end when she came to see us. She had just been called into the principal's office because of her frequent temper flare-ups in class. She feared she might lose her position.

Although Jennifer *thought* she was eating a healthy diet, when we discussed what she typically ate, we discovered that she consumed mostly high calcium foods. Because her symptoms were so severe, we suggested that she start by both changing her diet and by taking vitamin-mineral supplements. While she was willing to add many high magnesium foods to her daily diet, she was unwilling to give up her "favorite foods." However, as she became more aware of the effects these foods, particularly bleached flour pastas, cheeses and high caffeine foods, she gradually began to eliminate them and pay more attention to preparing high magnesium foods for herself.

Initially her family wasn't willing to change their diet. They felt that something was wrong with "Mom" and it was *she* who had to change. So Jennifer had to continue fixing the families' regular meals. Jennifer soon recognized that having to prepare two entirely different types of diets each day made it especially hard for her. At times, under stress, she would fall back to her old eating patterns. During those times, she felt noticeably more irritable and returned to her "old grouchy self."

Even so, at the end of the first month, her ability to cope had improved significantly. Because she was unable to be consistent with her diet, she eventually chose to add natural progesterone to her treatment program. For a while, this worked very well for her. Within three months, she began to follow the diet consistently and was able to discontinue the progesterone. By the end of six months, she had to take the supplements only on those occasions when she went off of her diet.

When we last heard from Jennifer, she was entirely symptom-free and her family had begun to eat the same way she did. Jennifer reported a great improvement in her home life as well as in her relationship with her students and her principal.

NOTE: If you find yourself being resistant this is perfectly OK. We realize that the changes we are asking you to make are not just simple and easy dietary changes. They are indeed life style changes. Not only how you eat will be affected, but also how you think, how you feel, how you shop, where you shop, how you feed your family and how they react to you.

We realize you may feel conflict about making many of the dietary changes we suggest and that it will also take you a while to reorganize your thinking and your eating habits. We know from our experience, personal and professional, that it is all well worth it.

We will be patient with you, if you will be patient with yourself. Start slowly. Start by adding more high magnesium/vitamin B6 foods to your diet and if you have severe PMS start by taking a well balanced anti-PMS vitamin-mineral supplement such as Metamorphosis, Women's Formula I. Remember, while this may not be the complete answer, it is an excellent first step and this will be a good start. Ultimately, though, if you want total control over the quality of your life, you will need to consider that the very best way you can regain full control is by carefully choosing the foods you eat by how they work for you. Remembering once again, "What you used to eat in the past caused your PMS, and what you choose to eat in the future can eliminate your PMS completely."

BASIC AND ADVANCED PMS ELIMINATION PROGRAMS

We have divided the remainder of this chapter into three sections:

Section I – Basic PMS Diet for Minimal or Mild PMS
Section II – Advanced PMS Diet for Moderate to Severe Sufferers of PMS
Section III – The 30-Day To No More PMS Program

SECTION I

BASIC PMS DIETARY PROGRAM

If you only suffer from very minimal to mild PMS you are probably already eating a basically good diet, or your system still has sufficient reserves of magnesium and vitamin B6, or you do not ha e a genetic tendency to have severe PMS.

It is very likely that you will need only small modifications to your existing diet to become symptom free. For you we offer our very simple, easy to use Basic PMS Diet Program. Read it through and make the necessary changes and you should do very well. If you do not, you can either use a good PMS vitamin-mineral supplement such as our Metamorphosis, Women's Formula I, to give you the boost you need to become symptom free rapidly– even within 30 days.

If this still does not do the job than read Section II, the Advanced PMS Dietary Program and make whatever changes you need to make to become symptom free.

Once you are entirely free for a period of 6 months than you can use the Basic PMS Diet as your long term Maintenance Diet.

Whether you use the Advanced Diet Program or not, the basic Dietary Program is still the basic nutritional treatment program for PMS so read it through thoroughly, understand it, and use what works for you.

A DIETARY PROGRAM TO ELIMINATE PREMENSTRUAL SYNDROME (PMS)

We have repeatedly stressed that we believe PMS is a condition created by a number of specific dietary deficiencies, magnesium and vitamin B6, and worsened by an excess of certain other foods and nutrients, such as refined and processed foods, simple sugars, large amounts of calcium and moderate to large amounts of caffeine in your diet act together to create PMS and its symptoms. When deficiencies of magnesium and vitamin B6 are combined with excesses of refined sugar, caffeine they not only create PMS, but also worsen it once it already exists.

PMS and many of the other estrogen excess syndromes will clearly respond and improve to a substantial decrease in circulating estrogen which was produced by the dietary deficiencies which initially created the PMS syndrome. Once a PMS woman begins to eat an anti-PMS diet, one which is exactly right for her and her bodily needs, she will find that her PMS symptoms will soon disappear and that the other medical-gynecologic conditions caused by excess estrogens will also tend to begin to resolve.

In the end, a treatment program consisting of diet that can reverse the specific problems that have caused your PMS is the very safest, easiest and most productive way to treat your PMS. It is in a sense correcting the very cause of the imbalances that lead to the clinical signs, symptoms and anatomical abnormalities we call PMS. On top of this how can you go wrong eating a good, sound, healthy diet. Many years ago we adopted the following motto, "It was what you ate that caused you to have PMS and now it is what you eat that will help you eliminate your PMS." In this section we hope to provide insight into how you can make the necessary changes and the foods you can now pick from.

The primary treatment of PMS therefore should be the reversal of the dietary deficiencies and excesses which originally cause it. This can be done most simply by adopting a diet of whole healthy foods, eliminating refined and processed foods and finally when needed, adding foods which are high in magnesium and the B vitamins into the healthy, whole food diet. In certain situations where women have severe PMS or wish very rapid results adding special balanced vitamin-mineral supplements and by carefully reducing and eliminating the intake of those foods which stimulate PMS, such as foods high in calcium, caffeine, refined sugars and processed foods, PMS can be controlled, reduced and even eliminated.

WHAT THEN DO I NEED TO DO TO INCREASE MAGNESIUM IN MY DIET AND REDUCE CALCIUM, CAFFEINE AND REFINED AND PROCESSED SUGARS?

The first step is to change your diet and begin the process of eliminating, as much as you can, all processed and refined foods from your daily diet. This will be covered in a separate section on recognizing and eliminating processed and refined food later within this chapter. The next step is to begin to choose and eat a basic whole healthy foods diet. This too will be covered in a separate section later in this Basic and Advanced PMS Diets and Appendix B. The third step is to learn which foods are high in magnesium and the B vitamins and then begin adding these foods to your daily diet. The last step for women with severe or resistant PMS symptoms is to learn which foods are high in calcium, caffeine and refined and processed sugars and then begin a steady process of eliminating these foods. Once again you can find out which foods are high in calcium and caffeine and refined sugars later on in this chapter in Tables 5, 7 and 8, and in Appendix E Caffeine Content of Foods. Basically this means is that you will be eating more natural and whole foods just like you grandparents and great-grandparents did, food will taste better and you will be feeding your body a much higher grade of fuel. It also means eating less processed and refined foods, such as foods in cans, boxes or frozen foods and more whole, fresh foods. The benefits from a whole, fresh food diet is astronomical as many of the most common medical problems today coronary heart disease, stroke, high blood pressure, obesity, diabetes and even arthritis have all been linked to a poor diet and experts now recommend that prevention from this conditions is best started by eating basically the exact same diet we are suggesting her...."a good healthy diet."

The dietary program we are about to provide to you can do all of this for you, it can help you to eliminate your PMS, reduce your risk of coronary heart disease, stroke, high blood pressure, obesity, diabetes and arthritis. The benefits of this type of eating exceed eliminating PMS, this same diet can provide an abundance of vitamins and minerals and micro nutrients that can also strengthen your immune system, reduce blood cholesterol levels, increase vitality and help your healing processes. It is basically the same diet that experts are now recommending for preventing cancer, gout, for safe weight loss, and for life-extension.

In the following list healthy foods we have listed the foods in each section with the highest magnesium levels first and going down to those with lower levels of magnesium for each food listed. You can also use Figure F as a general guide to picking your foods for this list.

THE PMS ELIMINATION DIET:

A) **Meat - Protein Group**: *Eat two to three - 4 ounces - servings each day.* Meat, fish and foul should be weighed raw, all fat and bone should be removed before cooking. Most supermarkets will cut and package meats in 4 ounce, boneless, skinless and fat trimmed portions ready for the freezer. Another hint is to have your butcher put wax paper between each slice so that you can separate each slice of meat and package them individually.

You may select your protein from the following:

Beef: Round steak, bottom roast, tenderloin steak, brisket, pot roast-arm
Veal: Veal leg
Lamb: All cuts
Game Meats: Duck, pheasant, antelope, elk, buffalo, moose, deer
Pork: Pork chops, loin roast or canned ham
Chicken: The leg, drumstick, thigh, breast

Turkey: Breast meat

Fish and Seafood: Pollack, fresh white tuna or packed in water, swordfish, bluefish, salmon, sea bass, cod, bass, imitation crab, sole, yellowtail, turbot, mackerel, rockfish-rock cod, oysters, monkfish, halibut, grouper, abalone, white fish, haddock, red snapper, shad, trout, halibut, orange roughy, catfish, shrimp, lobster, crayfish, clams, mussels, scallops.

Egg White: While not particularly high in magnesium provided an excellent form of protein. The white can either be separated from an egg or eaten as egg replacer from the market.

If you are a vegetarian or do not wish to have animal protein you can substitute 4 oz. portions of defatted soy protein such as Tofu, beans and whole grained rice eaten together, or you can use an approved protein shake. Vegetarians can avoid meat products entirely and we will help you to create an all vegetarian meal plan, if you contact us.

The Following Meats Should Be Eaten Only Occasionally:
Herring, salmon, liver, ribs, and other fattier cuts of meat as they are higher in fat and increase your risk of cardiovascular disease. Read about cheese and dairy products below.

B) **Bread/Grain/Seeds Group**: ***Eat AT LEAST three or more servings each day.***
One serving equals one slice or portion: Rye Crisp (natural, seasoned or sesame), Rye Snacks, brown rice cake, brown rice-millet cakes, brown rice-buckwheat cakes, Melba Toast, Whole Wheat cakes or low calorie bread sticks by Keebler or one slice of any 30 to 50 calorie whole grain breads. You may also have ½ cup of cooked wild rice (again 30-50 calories per ½ cup of cooked wild rice). Wasa Golden Rye or Multigrain crackers can also be used. Read labels to evaluate total fat content (see section of Reading Labels).

Breakfast cereals can be quite valuable both as a meal for breakfast and as snacks during the day to quickly raise magnesium levels. Nutri Grain corn cereal, wheat germ-toasted, Grape Nuts, 100% Bran, Ralston Flakes, Puffed Wheat-plain (without sugar), Wheatena-cooked, Post Bran flakes, Bran Buds, Ralston-cooked, All Bran, Bran Chex, Natural Bran Flakes, King Vitaman, Puffed Rice-plain, Shredded Wheat Biscuits-plain, Oat bran,-cooked, Kellogg Corn Flakes, Roman Meal-cooked, Kellogg Raisin Bran, Kellogg Bran Flakes, Nutri Grain Rye, Post Raisin Bran, Wheat Chex, Oatmeal-cooked, Post Grapenuts Flakes, Quaker Oat Bran, Nutri Grain Wheat, Rice Krispies, Special K

Grains in general are high in magnesium. The following are the highest and can be used in breads, cereals and in cooking in general. Corn, Rice Bran, cornmeal, popcorn, millet, rice cakes (above), Rice and Buckwheat cakes, corn grits, cornnuts, corn flour, buckwheat groats (whole or flour), wild rice, brown rice, Bulgur, Rye Flour, Trititicale flour and whole grain, Wheat (whole grain, whole grain flour, hard wheat, Durham wheat, sprouted wheat, semolina), barley, oats and oat bran, soba noodles, soy flour, potato flour, couscous.

Many seeds and nuts are also high in magnesium. The following are highest and can be used during the week to two weeks before the onset of menstruation to help raise magnesium levels quickly. Pumpkin and squash seeds, cashews, peanuts and peanut butter, chestnuts, pecans, walnuts, mixed dry nuts, sunflower seeds, macadamia nuts, pistachio nuts, filberts. Flavored nuts are okay, but nuts which have sugar or honey on them should be avoided. If you have elevated triglycerides -fats in the blood, use only dry roasted nuts and only when necessary to quickly raise magnesium levels during the PMS period.

The Following Should Be Avoided:
Cookies, cakes, donuts, bagels, breads baked with white flours, sugar or fats such as butter, lard. Crisco™ or other shortening products.

C) **Fruit Group**: *Eat AT LEAST two to four servings each day.*
No size limits on servings*: plantains, banana and banana flakes, passion fruits, avocado, peaches, carambola, lychees, nectarines, pineapple, plums, casaba melon, acerola, grapefruit, melon balls, fruit cocktail, oranges and orange juice, watermelon, apples, persimmons, apricots, guava, lemons, pears, tangerines, cantaloupe, and honeydew are all okay as are any berries including strawberries, raspberries, boysenberries or blueberries and grapes.

D) **Complex Carbohydrate - Vegetable Group**: *You should eat AT LEAST three to five 1 cup each serving of vegetables each day.* They may be eaten raw, lightly steamed, cooked alone or combination. Vegetables, especially those listed in Group I below, are considered "free" foods and large quantities may be eaten as part of meals or as a snack between meals. Not only are vegetables helpful in satisfying hunger, they are also high in vitamins, minerals, enzymes and fiber.

Group I - You May Eat *All You Want* of The Following Vegetables:
The following are high in magnesium and should be eaten often in some combination*. Corn, potatoes, navy beans, beets, succotash, black beans, mung bean sprouts, ginger root, tomato (fresh, cooked, stewed, puree, Italian and Mexican), tomatillo, cowpeas, eggplant, water

chestnuts, lima beans, mushrooms (all types), seaweed-Irish moss, peppers (Bell, red, green, sweet, jalapeno), lentils, squash (butternut, Italian, summer, winter or zucchini), taro and poi.

Group II - Eat Only Occasionally an in the Non-PMS Part of Your Cycle:
The following are relatively low in magnesium and, while quite healthy and good for you, should be combined with one or more high magnesium foods when eaten. Amaranth, rugula, asparagus, alfalfa sprouts, bamboo shoots, beet greens, broccoli,

brussels sprouts, bean sprouts, cabbage, cress. cauliflower, celery, chard, chilies (green, pepperoncini, red, yellow), Chinese mixed vegetables (canned by LaChoy), chop suey vegetables (LaChoy), chrysanthemum leaves, chives, collard greens, cucumbers, dandelion greens, endive, escarole, garlic, jicama, kale, kohlrabi, leek, lettuce (all types), lotus root, mustard greens, okra, onions, parsley, pea pods, pickles (all types), pimento, radishes, radicchio, rutabagas, sauerkraut, shallots, soy bean sprouts, spinach, green snap beans, string beans, turnips and watercress.

E) Eliminate Foods Which Are High in Caffeine

These include coffee, teas, chocolate, soft drinks, Aspirin with caffeine, etc. Caffeine promotes and worsens PMS. It is important to read labels of everything you purchase to see if ti contains caffeine. Substitute decaf coffee, herbal teas and caffeine fress soft drinks. See Appendix E for List Caffeine Content in Common Foods.

EIGHT IMPORTANT POINTS YOU MUST BE AWARE OF:

1) **Dairy Should Only Be Used Occasionally and Always in Moderation!**
   Dairy products (milk, cheese, yogurt, cream, mild shakes) are high in calcium and hence will promote and worsen PMS. It is important to eat or drink products in strict moderation and only during the non-PMS portion of the menstrual cycle. When eaten dairy products should be used as part of the protein part of the diet (see Meats - Protein Group above) For the best results use only low fat, skim milk, cottage cheese, Provolone and other skim milk cheeses, i.e., goat cheeses are lower in both fat and cholesterol and can be eaten safely on a periodic basis but only in small portions less than ½ cup per serving and once again best during the non-PMS portion of your cycle. No high fat/high cholesterol dairy products are suggested on this diet. Vitamins and supplements can be used if your daily intake of dairy is significantly restricted. (You may take a magnesium/calcium supplement, if you wish to maximize effects of

Ca there should be 2 Magnesium for each Calcium unit.)

2) **Simple Carbohydrates Should Be Eliminated or Restricted!**
Simple carbohydrates are essentially any processed and refined foods. They promote and worsen PMS. These foods are usually packaged or pre-prepared and found in dry form in boxes or TV-type dinners. These foods are not only processed but often also high in fat content. It is also suggested to eat a minimum of foods such as white rice, white-bleached-flour breads and other white processed flour products, macaroni, white-flour spaghetti and noodles. These foods deplete magnesium which is essential for their metabolism and for its role in reducing atherosclerotic heart and vascular diseases. Also all baked goods (except those listed above) as they are pure starch as well as high in fat or lard, and hence, very fattening.

We also suggest restricting, as much as possible, all forms of processed sugars. This includes, but not limited to, white table sugar, turbinado sugar, brown sugar, molasses, corn sweetener, corn syrup, corn starch and modified food starches also as we suggested above white flour and white rice, processed mashed potatoes. Often the only way you will know whether these substances are in foods is to read the label on the package or can. Of course, cookies, cakes and pies are also to be avoided. This also includes supposed low calorie foods such as Weight Watchers, Stouffer's, Health Gourmet and others, etc. Often the only way you will know what is in the foods you would like to eat is to *read the labels* on the packages or cans. Of course, certain foods such as cookies, cakes, donuts and pies you already know are not good for you.

Sugar Found in Foods in the Following Forms

White table sugar, turbinado sugar, brown sugar, honey, molasses, corn sweetener, corn syrup, any foods which may end in -ose: fructose, dextrose, maltose, dextro-maltose or malto-dextrose, barley sweetener, corn starch and modified food starches, alcohol, white flour, bleached flour, white rice, rice flour, rice vinegar and rice sweetener and processed mashed potatoes.

Table 5

3) **Alcoholic Beverages Are Not Allowed!**
Alcohol is basically pure sugar and therefore, should be strictly avoided all through the month, however this is especially important in the week or so before PMS symptoms would start. Any use of alcohol will disrupt, slow down or destroy your ability to maintain blood sugar control and control your PMS.

4) **Avoid And Eliminate Fat Whenever You Can.**
Our intention here is not just to help you eliminate your PMS but also to present you with a good and healthy dietary program. Eliminating fat in the diet helps you to control your weight, and decrease your ultimate risk of coronary heart disease (atherosclerosis). If you eat meats, it is extremely important that you trim off all visible skin and fat from your meat, fish or foul before cooking them. We also suggest that you do not fry foods in oil. If you wish to fry your foods, use PAM or a Teflon™ or other non-stick frying pan. It is also helpful to stop using butter and margarine in or on your foods. To help eliminate fat from meats and fish we recommend that you cook items by broiling on a rack so that cooked-liquid fats can drop off of the meats into a tray below and be discarded, however, baking and boiling are also acceptable. Egg yolk is high in fat and should be avoided. Once again please read the section on Reading Labels in this document. You may use olive oil, canola or safflower oil on salads or in your cooking. These oils when used in small amounts can actually lower serum cholesterol.

5) **Drink Plenty of Water!**
Patients should drink at least 8 large (8 oz.) glasses - equivalent to 64 ounces - of water a day. By drinking plenty of water, low-sugar beverages, tea (preferably Herbal) and decaffeinated coffee, you can avoid constipation, dehydration and ketosis. The juice of one lemon should be included in your daily fluid intake. Instead of that cup of coffee in the morning, boil some water and squeeze the lemon juice into it. An artificial sweetener can be added to reduce the tartness. Remember not to use sodas, even diet sodas as your only source of fluids.

6) **Physical Activity Is a Must!**
Physical activity is essential. Many studies show that women who exercise regularly have much fewer problems with PMS. An increase in activity helps keep both your appetite and weight down. Physical exercise not only burns' fat but it mobilizes water, maintains flexibility, decreases risks of heart disease and osteoporosis and much more. Dedicate yourself to making physical activity a part of your life's routine and enjoy the benefits!

7) **No Junk Food Snacking!**

Junk food snacking can slow your progress down, promote and worsen PMS and can be your downfall! So no snacking. Most junk foods are refined and processed foods, are high in refined sugars, salt and white flours. They neither are healthy nor do they help in any way to eliminate PMS, if fact they will more often than not worsen existing PMS. Eat three to four small meals a day. Always think before eating. As we just said, most junk foods have significant amounts of refined flours, starches, animal fats, refined sugars or additives and preservatives which are not very healthy and promote and worsen PMS. When you control your appetite, you control your blood sugar and your weight. If you are hungry in-between meals, eat as much of the low-calorie free vegetables you wish. You can also eat a portion from your fruit or the bread-grain group as a mid-morning, mid-afternoon or late night snack. Fluids, water with lemon, low calorie sodas, herbal tea or decaf coffee will also reduce cravings. You can however, use nuts, seeds, popcorn, fruit and vegetables from the Group I list, as snacks or possibly better small meals.

8) **Avoid Hypoglycemia (Low Blood Sugar)**

Some people may find that they are having episodes of dizziness, sweating, slight or moderate confusion, difficulty thinking and concentrating or even a rapid pulse somewhere between 3 to 6 hours after eating. This might be due to low blood sugar. This can be controlled by eating 4 to 6 small meals a day. This is done by dividing up the total of what is to be eaten over the day into 4 to 6 small portions. Often if episodes of hypoglycemia are mild, your fruit or bread-grain servings can be used as small meal portions between meals (see item 7 above).

TEN USEFUL TIPS

1) Spices, herbs, seasonings and condiments are allowed and even encouraged. Take this opportunity to discover and experiment with new seasonings - be they mild and earthy or zesty and exciting! By using distinctive flavors and aromas, you decrease monotony and increase interest. Salt may be used moderately. Avoid those products which have oil (other than olive oil, canola or safflower oil), alcohol or sugar added to them.

2) Avoid caffeine, if at all possible. Caffeine is a stimulant and as we stated above it can promote and worsen PMS. First, caffeine can cause some very unusual problems such as anxiety or panic attacks and irregular heart beat (palpitations). Secondly, caffeine is often used to decrease hunger, however, it is not very effective because as it wears off hunger returns and is often

3) If your weight is an issue then for salads use a **Low-Calorie No-Fat Salad Dressing**. Make sure it contains little or no oils or dairy products. Fresh lemon juice, black pepper and sweet basil make a good salad dressing. Consider eating fresh vegetables' raw. This has several benefits.

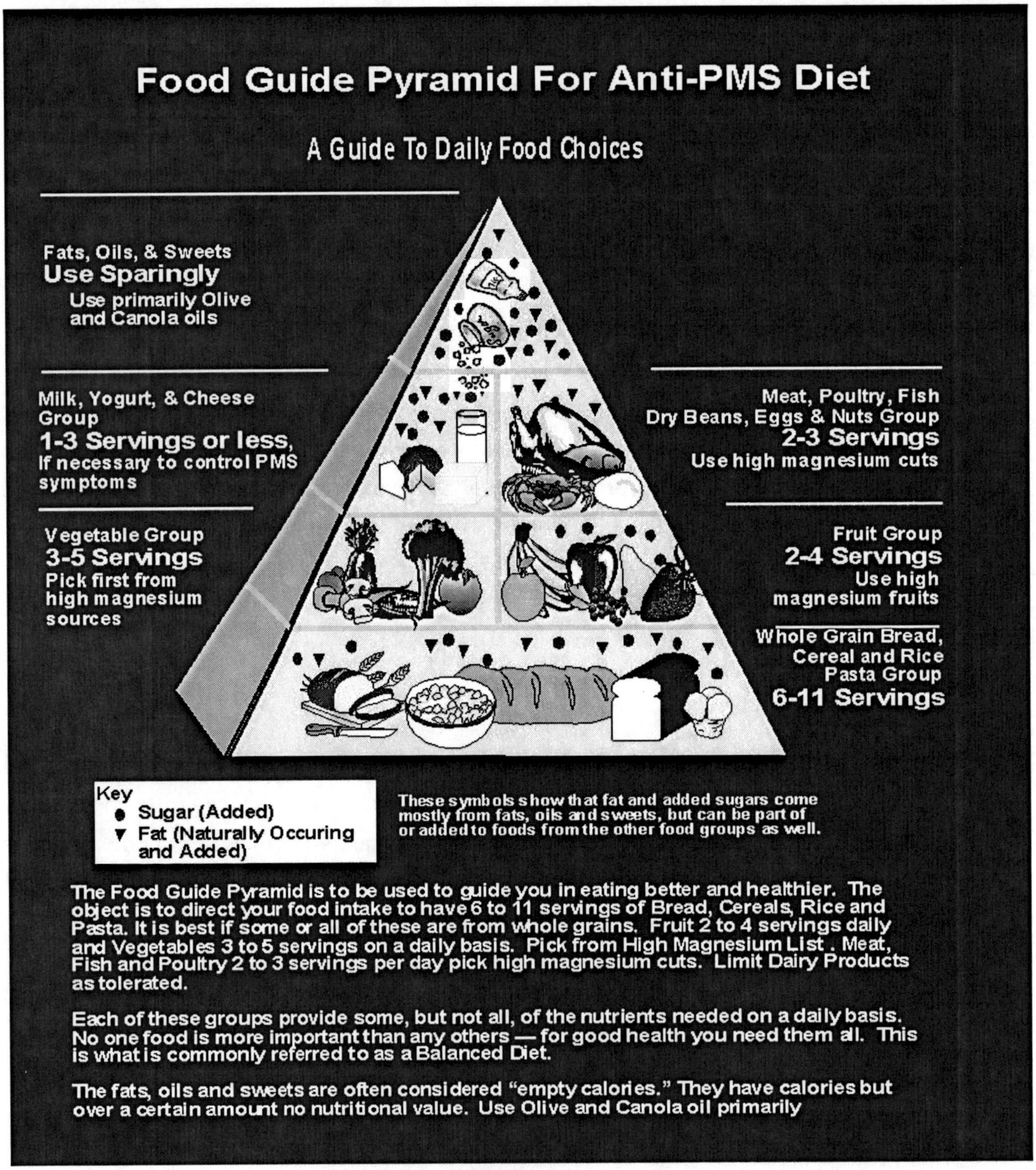

Figure F

Figure F text:

Food Guide Pyramid For Anti-PMS Diet

A Guide To Daily Food Choices

Fats, Oils, & Sweets **Use Sparingly** Use primarily Olive and Canola oils

Milk, Yogurt, & Cheese Group **1-3 Servings or less,** If necessary to control PMS symptoms

Vegetable Group **3-5 Servings** Pick first from high magnesium sources

Meat, Poultry, Fish Dry Beans, Eggs & Nuts Group **2-3 Servings** Use high magnesium cuts

Fruit Group **2-4 Servings** Use high magnesium fruits

Whole Grain Bread, Cereal and Rice Pasta Group **6-11 Servings**

Key
● Sugar (Added)
▼ Fat (Naturally Occuring and Added)

These symbols show that fat and added sugars come mostly from fats, oils and sweets, but can be part of or added to foods from the other food groups as well.

The Food Guide Pyramid is to be used to guide you in eating better and healthier. The object is to direct your food intake to have 6 to 11 servings of Bread, Cereals, Rice and Pasta. It is best if some or all of these are from whole grains. Fruit 2 to 4 servings daily and Vegetables 3 to 5 servings on a daily basis. Pick from High Magnesium List. Meat, Fish and Poultry 2 to 3 servings per day pick high magnesium cuts. Limit Dairy Products as tolerated.

Each of these groups provide some, but not all, of the nutrients needed on a daily basis. No one food is more important than any others — for good health you need them all. This is what is commonly referred to as a Balanced Diet.

The fats, oils and sweets are often considered "empty calories." They have calories but over a certain amount no nutritional value. Use Olive and Canola oil primarily

First, you are no longer attached to salad dressings. Secondly, it is a treat for those who like natural flavors. If you do feel that you want an oil dressing every once in a while use olive, canola or safflower oils only.

4) If you normally eat very fast and therefore often overeat, try the following: Before eating drink a full 8 oz. glass of water. You can add lemon (one slice or a whole squeezed lemon) if you like. This will help to fill you up so you're not tempted to overeat.

5) To aid digestion and slow your eating and keep you from overeating. Chew your food slowly and completely the longer you take the longer it will take to eat. This solves two problems: Often we eat so fast that our brain doesn't have time to register that we have eaten. The better you chew your food the easier it is to digest it. Count 8 to 10 chews per mouthful of food. This will help to reduce overeating.

6) Never eat when you are feeling stressed. When you feel stressed, you tend to eat too fast. Also during the process of stress blood is directed away from the digestive system, hence the ability of your body to properly digest the food you have just eaten is reduced.

7) As best as is possible, try to eat at about the same time every day. This not only allows the body to anticipate eating but it allows you to more effectively use appetite suppressants or prepare adequate nutritional aids and supplements.

8) Do not eat *immediately* before or after exercising. Once again digestion can be hampered and the end result is increased hunger and less effective assimilation of nutrients. It is always best to exercise first wait 15-30 minutes and then eat. If you do this you will raise your metabolic rate and maximize digestion as well as the nutritional value of your food while also maximizing fat utilization.

9) If you are having digestive problems consider eating along the lines of the Food Hygiene method. This means eating only from fruit, vegetable or bread-grain groups for breakfast and lunch and then meats and other proteins later for dinner. If you wish information about this concept please let us know and we will work with you to prepare a program especially for you.

10) Be smart about calories. Be smart about cooking, Be smart about what and how you eat. And be smart about exercise.

WATER HELPS KEEP FAT AWAY AND KEEP YOU HYDRATED AND HEALTHY

It sounds almost too simple, but drinking at least eight 8-ounce glasses of water a day helps keep the fat away. Water naturally suppresses the appetite and helps your body metabolize stored fat.
The kidneys can't function properly without enough water and when that happens the overload is dumped onto the liver. One of the liver's functions is to metabolize fat into usable energy for the body. But if the liver has to do some of the kidney's work it can't operate at full throttle, and as a result more fat remains stored in then blood fat levels rise and this makes cardiovascular disease harder to prevent, and blood sugar harder to control.

Drinking water is the best thing for fluid retention. When the body gets less water, it perceives this as a threat to survival and begins to hold on to every drop. The best way to beat water retention is to give your body what it needs - plenty or water. Only then will stored water be released.

If you have an excess problem with water retention, salt may be the culprit. Your body will tolerate sodium only in a certain concentration. The more salt you eat, the more water your system retains to dilute it. Drinking water takes away the excess sodium by forcing it through the kidneys.

Water also helps maintain proper muscle tone by giving muscles their natural ability to contract. Along with exercise, water helps prevent skin from sagging and looking old before your time. Water plumps up the skin and leaves it clear, healthy and resilient.

Water helps rid the body of waste. Water is necessary to flush metabolic waste. Water helps relieve constipation and encourages normal bowel function.

How much water is enough? Like we said, eight 8-ounce glasses every day. But the overweight person should drink more water than the thin one. The overweight person should drink an additional glass for every 25 pounds of excess fat. The amount you drink should also be increased if you exercise briskly or if the weather is hot and dry.

Section II

ADVANCED PMS DIET

This section is for women who suffer from moderate to severe PMS. They need much more dietary help. Start by reading through the Basic PMS Dietary Program, next get started on a good PMS vitamin-mineral supplement such as the Metamorphosis, Women's Formula I. Read Section II carefully and follow the steps outlined there until you become symptoms free. The first thing you will need to know is how to use the Desired Foods (Foods to Be Eaten) and foods To Be Avoided (offender Foods) Lists.

USING THE FOODS TO BE EATEN AND FOODS TO AVOID LISTS

The next step is to look through the "Foods To Be Eaten" or "Desired Foods"- High Magnesium Foods List Table 7) and then the Foods to Be Avoided List (Table 8). In the Foods to Be Eaten List, familiarize yourself with the foods that are highest in magnesium and vitamin B6. Since, interestingly enough, most foods high in magnesium are also high in B6, picking good foods should be quite simple. As you familiarize yourself with the foods on this High Magnesium Foods List, notice how many of them you eat frequently. If you notice there are quite a few foods you eat and enjoy, then it is more likely that your PMS problems may be caused by a relative deficiency problem.

In this case, you will need to evaluate your diet for excess calcium, simple carbohydrates and caffeine. With the data we have already given, you should now be able to quickly determine which types of foods will relieve and which types of foods will worsen your symptoms. Now make your own lists of good and not so good foods based on this new criterion. Use the list we have provided as well as any other reliable sources you have at your command.

If you find that you don't like or rarely eat many of the foods from the High Magnesium Foods List, then it is likely you have an absolute deficiency. In this case, start by choosing as many high magnesium foods as you can, then work them into your meal plan.

MAGNESIUM TO CALCIUM RATIO

It is in your best interest to eat every three to four hours (at least six small meals each day). Each small meal or snack should have a high magnesium food so that you have a relatively constant flow of magnesium into your system throughout the day. Your goal is to create meals and menus which allow at least twice as many milligrams of magnesium as calcium, that is, preferably a 2 to 1 ratio of magnesium to calcium, in your daily diet.

To maintain this 2 to 1 ratio throughout the day, pick at least one food which is high in magnesium and low in calcium for each meal. You can also use the High Magnesium Foods List to make sure that you are taking in at least 300 to 600 milligrams of magnesium daily.

It is important that you start this process slowly for magnesium (as in Milk of Magnesia) is an exceptionally good laxative. Large amounts of magnesium can cause loose bowel movements and even diarrhea. If you start slowly, your system will soon adjust to the increasing amounts of magnesium you take in each day. A side benefit (or problem) of this diet is that most people who maximize magnesium in their diets soon find that they are having a normal bowel movement at least once daily and in many cases, after each meal. Actually, this is the normal state for a healthy individual. Much to our detriment, the Great American Diet which is low in fiber, low in magnesium and high in simple refined carbohydrates and processed foods often leaves us constipated.

The reason we suggest you make sure that your overall daily intake of magnesium is greater than 300 milligrams (mg) is that diets containing less than this amount may not be sufficient to relieve your symptoms. The RDA (Recommended Daily Allowance) of magnesium is at least 400 mg daily. Therefore we strongly suggest that, if you can, your diet should contain more than 300 and even possibly as high as 600 mg or more of magnesium each day.

This amount is considered perfectly safe as magnesium toxicity does not occur until dosages reach 2,000 mg or more daily. It has been our experience that diarrhea occurs long before toxicity which would make it virtually impossible to get an excess of magnesium. If you go higher than 400 mg of magnesium daily you can afford to be more permissive in the amount of calcium you take in. In this case, as always, use your symptoms as a guide. If your symptoms get worse, you should increase high magnesium foods and decrease the high calcium foods in your diet. The same, of course, is true for the other offender foods. As symptoms decrease and disappear you will know that you are getting closer to the diet that works best and is the most healthful for you.

As you look at the Foods to Avoid List, you will probably notice immediately that this list is considerably larger than the High Magnesium Foods List. This, of course, is one of the reasons why PMS exists. There are naturally many more high calcium foods than high magnesium foods.

You should also notice that this list is set up differently than the High Magnesium Foods List. In the Foods to Avoid Lists we have listed the amount of calcium in each food first. We placed those highest in calcium at the top of the list. Each succeeding entry contains correspondingly less calcium and more magnesium. This is so that you can see at a glance which foods are higher in calcium. In the High Magnesium Foods List, the amount of magnesium in each food comes first, with the highest amount of magnesium at the top of the list. The foods on the Foods to Avoid List are the ones to be minimized or eliminated during the Premenstrual phase.

Eventually, you will reach a list labeled, Neutral Foods. The foods on this list all have ratios of magnesium to calcium between 1:1 and 2:1. These foods are not significantly higher in either magnesium or calcium. Unless your symptoms are extremely difficult to manage, you can include all you want of these foods in your recipes, menus or meals. They will neither worsen nor improve your symptoms. If your symptoms are very fragile and you are having difficulty managing them, it's probably best to use more of the foods from the High Magnesium Foods list and select these foods instead of others which are either neutral or high in calcium.

All three lists, Desired Foods - High Magnesium Foods (Table 6), Foods to Avoid - High Calcium Foods (Table 7) and Neutral Foods (Table 8), as well as Meats, Poultry and Fish List (Table 9) show not only the specific amounts of magnesium and calcium but also the ratios of magnesium to calcium (M g/Ca). We have added these ratios for your convenience as they can provide you with an instant way of evaluating each food and determining whether it will give you the proper ratio for your diet. You will, hopefully, notice that throughout the lists the ratios do not take into consideration the total amount of each substance. For example, one food might have 4 milligrams of magnesium and 2 milligrams of calcium. The ratio of this food will therefore be 2:1 Mg/Ca. Another food may have 200 milligrams of magnesium and 100 milligrams of calcium. Its Mg/Ca ratio will also be 2:1.

If a food has only 4 milligrams of magnesium and a second food has 200 milligrams magnesium, which foods do you think would be better for you? Both may be good foods, but each has a different amount of magnesium and calcium. If you need a larger amount of magnesium quickly then the 200 milligram food would be the one to choose. However, you will also get 100 milligrams of calcium with it. The first food has negligible amounts of both magnesium and calcium so you could essentially eat as much as you want without doing harm to yourself. The second food will not only raise your magnesium levels rapidly but also your calcium levels as well. However, with these foods you will not only maintain the Mg/Ca ratio, but you will also keep the calcium levels down.

> **Once You Learn How to Eat Correctly,
> You Can Essentially Eat Anything and Everything
> You Want and Still Be Able to Remain Symptom Free.**

Table 7

DESIRED FOODS – HIGH MAGNESIUM FOODS
FOODS TO BE EATEN AS OFTEN AS POSSIBLE

FOODS WITH HIGH MG/CA RATIO	MG	CA	MG/CA
FRUITS			
Banana, raw, 1 medium	33	7	4.7
Banana, dried, 1 oz.	132	32	4.1
Passion fruit (Purple Grandilla), raw 1 medium	5	2	2.5
FRUIT & VEGETABLE JUICES			
Passion fruit, yellow, fresh, 8 fl. oz.	41	9	4.6
Coconut, milk, canned, 1 cup	104	40	2.6
Coconut, milk, raw, 1 cup	89	39	2.3
VEGETABLES			
Mushrooms, shiitake, dried, 4	20	2	10.0
Avocado, Florida, 1 medium	104	33	5.5
Mushrooms, shiitake, cooked, 4	10	2	5.0
Potato, baked without skin, 1 medium	39	8	4.9
Potato, microwaved without skin, 1 medium	39	8	4.9
Avocado, California, 1 medium	70	19	3.7
Beets, boiled, ½ cup	31	9	3.4
Succotash, cooked, ½ cup	51	16	3.2

FOODS WITH HIGH MG/CA RATIO	MG	CA	MG/CA
Blackeyed peas (cow peas), dried, raw, ½ cup	230	75	3.1
Peas, green, dried, ½ cup	180	64	2.8
Peas, green, split, cooked, 1 cup	31	22	2.7
Potato, baked with skin, 1 medium	55	20	2.75
Potato, hash browns, homemade, 1 medium	16	6	2.7
Black beans, cooked, 1 cup	121	47	2.6
Lima beans, cooked or dried, 1 cup	82	32	2.6
Potato, boiled without skin, 1 medium	26	10	2.6
Sesame, kernel, toasted 1 Tablespoon	98	37	2.6
Ginger root, raw, ½ cup sliced	10	4	2.5
Mushrooms, cooked, ½ cup	10	4	2.5
Potato, microwaved with skin, 1 medium	54	22	2.5
Dock, raw or cooked, ½ cup	69	29	2.4
Pepper, sweet, raw or cooked, ½ cup	7	3	2.3
Cowpeas (Blackeyed peas), cooked, ½ cup	91	42	2.2

GRAINS, BREADS, PASTAS & CRACKERS			
Corn germ, EnerG Foods, 1 cup	672	Trace	672:1
Sweet corn, 1 ear	48	3	16.0
Corn meal, Quaker Enriched/Aunt Jemima, 1 cup	12	Trace	12.0
Millet, 3.5 oz.	162	20	8.1
Wheat bran, Quaker unprocessed, 2 Tablespoon	46	6	7.7
Wheat germ, toasted, ¼ cup (1 oz.)	91	13	7.0
Rice, wild, ½ cup	129	19	7.0
Rice flour, EnerG Foods, ½ cup	60	13	4.6
Wheat, whole grain, 1 cup	160	40	4.0
Oat bran, Quaker, 1/3 cup (1 oz.)	67	20	3.4
Barley, Scotch, 1 cup	34	11	3.1
Rye grain, whole, 1 cup	115	38	3.0
Oats, oatmeal, quick, 1/3 cup dry (2/3 cooked)	40	14	2.9
Brown rice, ½ cup	88	32	2.8
Rye Krisp Crackers, plain and seasoned, ¼ sq.	34	12	2.8
Macaroni, enriched, cooked (not cheese) 1 cup	25	11	2.3
Spaghetti, enriched, cooked, 1 cup	25	11	2.3
Barley, light pearl, 1 cup	37	16	2.3
Buckwheat, whole grain, 1 cup	229	114	2.0

FOODS WITH HIGH MG/CA RATIO	MG	CA	MG/CA
NUTS & SEEDS (All 1 ounce servings)			
Pinyon, pine nuts, dried	67	2	33.5
Pumpkin seeds	152	12	12.7
Watermelon seeds	146	15	9.7
Ginko nuts, raw	8	1	8.0
Cashew butter	73	12	6.1
Cashews, dry roasted	74	13	5.7
Cashews, raw	74	13	5.7
Peanut butter, smooth/creamy	28	5	5.6
Chestnuts, roasted	26	5	5.2
Ginko nuts, canned	5	1	5.0
Chestnuts, dried	39	8	4.9
Butter nuts, dried	67	15	4.5
Acorns, Raw	5	24	4.8
Water chestnuts, Chinese	39	8	4.8
Pecans, dry roasted	10	38	3.8
Pecans, dry roasted	38	10	3.8
Coconut meat, dried	26	7	3.7
Peanuts, dry roasted	206	59	3.5
Sunflower seeds, dried	100	33	3.3
Sesame kernels, toasted	98	37	2.6

Foods To Avoid - Foods High In Calcium

In this list we will deal with foods which are best avoided. The foods on this list are divided into two parts: (1) foods to be entirely avoided and (2) foods which can be considered relatively neutral. The foods in the first list, *Foods to Avoid*, are generally best avoided entirely, if possible, during the critical period of the menstrual cycle, that, is the two weeks prior to the onset of the menstrual period, the time when PMS symptoms are often at their worst. These foods will tend to stimulate PMS and make your symptoms worse. They are high in calcium and relatively low in magnesium. These foods have ratios less than 1.0. The smaller the ratio number the more calcium (also the less magnesium).

The foods in the second list can be considered *Neutral Foods*. That is, they are approximately equal in calcium and magnesium. They are best avoided if you can choose a food from the *Foods High in Magnesium* list. However, they are much better than the foods on the *Foods to Avoid* list. The foods on the *Neutral Foods* list have magnesium to calcium ratios between 1.0 and 2.0.

HOW TO USE THIS LIST

In this list, we have placed the calcium values first. Foods on this list are ordered from the least desirable to the most desirable. At the top are those foods which have the lowest Mg/Ca ratio. The entries steadily increase toward those foods which are highest in their Mg/Ca ratio. This is only to allow you to visualize the relative amounts of calcium to magnesium. The numbers to the far right on this list still represent the ratio of magnesium to calcium (Mg/Ca). As the numbers increase, the relative amounts of magnesium increases and the foods become less of a problem.

The reader should take note as to how many more high calcium foods there are than high magnesium foods. It may become much more obvious as to why PMS is such a common problem in our society. We usually suggest that each woman make a list of the 10 most common foods she eats and note how many of them are likely to be foods which are high in calcium rather than magnesium. If you do this for yourself, we believe that you will certainly be able to see why you have PMS.

Table 8

FOODS TO AVOID - HIGH CALCIUM FOODS

FOODS WITH HIGH MG/CA RATIO	MG	CA	MG/CA
FRUITS			
Kumquats, raw, 1 medium	31	.31	0.01
Orange, Valencia, 1 medium	48	12	0.25
Orange, Naval, 1 medium	56	15	0.26
Crabapple, raw, 1 cup slices	20	7	0.35
Currants, red and white, raw, ½ cup	18	7	0.40
Gooseberry, raw, 1 cup	38	15	0.40
Grapes, American, raw, 1 cup	13	5	0.40
Papaya, raw, 1 medium	72	31	0.40
Fig, raw, 1 medium	18	8	0.40
Fig, dried, 10	269	111	0.40
Currants, black, European, raw, ½ cup	31	14	0.45
Mulberries, raw, 1 cup	55	25	0.45

FOODS WITH HIGH MG/CA RATIO	MG	CA	MG/CA
Pear, fresh, 1 medium	19	9	0.47
Grapes, European, raw, 1 cup	17	10	0.47
Apricot, fresh, 3 medium	15	8	0.50
Guava, raw, 1 medium	18	9	0.50
Cherry, red sour, canned, water pack, ½ cup	13	7	0.54
Boysenberries, frozen, 1 cup, unsweetened	36	21	0.58
Apple, whole with skin medium	10	6	0.60
Blackberries, raw, ½ cup	23	14	0.60
Cranberries, raw, 1 cup, whole	7	5	0.70
Quince, raw, 1 medium	10	7	0.70
Raisins, seedless, 2/3 cup	49	33	0.70
Apple, pared, 1 medium	6	5	0.80
Blueberries, raw, ½ cup	9	7	0.80
Cherries, raw, 10	10	8	0.80
Guava, Strawberry, raw, 1 cup	52	14	0.80
Grapefruit, pink, red and white, ½ medium	13	10	0.80
Loganberry, frozen, 1 cup	38	32	0.80
Loquats, raw, 10 medium	16	13	0.80
Raspberries, red, raw, 10	27	22	0.80
Strawberries, raw, 1 cup	21	16	0.80
Tangerine, raw, 1 medium	12	10	0.80
Prunes, cooked, ½ cup	24	21	0.87
Apple, dried, 10 rings	9	10	0.90
Mango, raw, 1 medium	21	18	0.90
Oheloberries, raw, 1 cup	10	9	0.90
Prune, dried, 10	43	38	0.90
Pear, dried, 10 halves	59	58	0.98

FRUIT & VEGETABLE JUICES			
Papaya, nectar, cooked, 8 fl. oz.	24	8	0.33
Pear, nectar, cooked, fl. oz.	11	6	0.54
Carrot, cooked, 6 fl. oz.	44	26	0.60
Pineapple, canned and frozen, 8 fl. oz.	42	34	0.80
Peach, nectar, cooked, 8 fl. oz.	13	11	0.85
Apple, frozen, concentrate, hydrated, 8 fl. oz.	14	12	0.86
Lemon, fresh, 8 fl. oz.	18	16	0.90

VEGETABLES			
Rhubarb, frozen, cooked, sweetened, 1 cup	174	15	0.08
Cabbage, Chinese, cooked, ½ cup	79	9	0.11

FOODS WITH HIGH MG/CA RATIO

FOODS WITH HIGH MG/CA RATIO	MG	CA	MG/CA
Garlic, raw, 3 cloves	16	2	0.13
Kale leaves, frozen, ½ cup chopped	90	12	0.13
Mustard greens, frozen, ½ cup chopped	75	10	0.13
Cress, Garden, 5-8 sprigs	81	11	0.14
Collard greens, frozen, ½ cup	179	26	0.15
Dandelion greens, raw, ½ cup chopped	52	10	0.20
Cabbage, Chinese, raw, ½ cup shredded	39	9	0.20
Watercress, raw, ½ cup chopped	20	4	0.20
Lettuce, Romaine, raw, ½ cup shredded	10	2	0.20
Turnip greens, cooked, ½ cup	125	21	0.20
Horseradish, 1 Tablespoon	28	7	0.25
Cabbage, green, raw, ½ cup shredded	16	5	0.30
Cabbage, red, raw, ½ cup shredded	18	5	0.30
Celery, raw or cooked, 1 stalk (7.5 inches long)	15	5	0.30
Chicory, greens, raw, ½ cup chopped	90	27	0.30
Endive (escarole), raw, ½ cup chopped	13	4	0.30
Parsley, raw, ½ cup chopped	39	13	0.30
Olives, green pickled, 2 medium	61	22	0.40
Onion, raw, cooked or dried, ½ cup chopped	20	08	0.40
Broccoli, cooked, frozen, ½ cup	47	19	0.40
Cauliflower, cooked, ½ cup	17	7	0.40
Sesame seeds, toasted and roasted, 1 oz.	281	101	0.40
Cabbage, cooked, ½ cup shredded	25	11	0.44
Turnip, ½ cup cubes	32	14	0.44
Broccoli, raw, ½ cup pieces	89	11	0.50
Cauliflower, raw, ½ cup pieces	14	7	0.50
Leek, raw, ¼ cup chopped	15	7	0.50
Lettuce, iceberg, 1 leaf	4	2	0.50
Rutabaga, cooked, ½ cup	36	18	0.50
Spinach, cooked, frozen, ½ cup	139	65	0.50
Tofu, firm, raw, ½ cup	258	118	0.50
Brussels sprouts, cooked, ½ cup (4 sprouts)	28	16	0.60
Carrots, cooked, ½ cup sliced	19	11	0.60
Carrots, raw, 1 medium	19	11	0.60
Pumpkin, cooked, ½ cup mashed	18	11	0.60
Snap beans, green/yellow, cooked, ½ cup	29	16	0.60
Squash, winter, baked, ½ cup cubed	14	8	0.60
Spinach, New Zealand, frozen, cooked, ½ cup	43	29	0.70
Sweet potato, baked, 1 medium	32	23	0.70
Kelp, 3.5 oz.	168	121	0.70

FOODS WITH HIGH MG/CA RATIO	MG	CA	MG/CA
Dulse, ½ cup	296	220	0.70
Kidney, red California beans, cooked, 1 cup	116	85	0.70
Potato, homemade mashed, ½ cup	27	19	0.70
Navy beans, cooked, 1 cup	128	107	0.80
Parsnip, cooked, ½ cup	29	23	0.80
Spinach, raw, ½ cup chopped	28	22	0.80
Asparagus, cooked, ½ cup (6 spears)	22	17	0.90
Alfalfa seed sprouts, raw, 1 cup	10	9	0.90
Chick peas (garbanzo beans), canned, 1 cup	78	70	0.90
Cucumber, raw, ½ cup sliced	7	6	0.90
French beans, cooked, 1 cup	111	99	0.90
Green peas, canned, ½ cup	17	15	0.90
Okra, cooked, ½ cup	50	46	0.90
Squash, summer, cooked, ½ cup sliced	24	22	0.90

GRAIN, BREAD & CRACKERS			
Hamburger buns, 1 roll	54	8	0.15
Hot dog buns, 1 roll	54	8	0.15
White bread, 1 slice	30	5	0.16
French bread, 1 slice	22	6	0.27
Pita bread, pita	31	10	0.30
Rye bread, American, 1 slice	20	6	0.30
Wheat bread, 1 slice	30	11	0.40
Bagels, 1 bagel	25	11	0.44
Saltine crackers, 2 crackers	4	2	0.50
Corn tortilla, 1 tortilla	42	20	0.50
Taco/tostada shell, 1 shell	16	11	0.70

NUTS & SEEDS (All 1 ounce servings)			
Walnuts, black	15	57	0.30
Mixed Nuts, dry roasted	20	64	0.30
Sesame, whole, roasted/toasted	281	101	0.40
Brazil Nuts, dried	64	50	0.80
Soy nuts, dry roasted, ½ cup	232	196	0.84
Filberts	209	184	0.90

Neutral Foods – How They Can Help Or Not

This is a third list, one we have not discussed up until now. If there are foods that you should eat and foods that you should not eat, then it is also likely that there are foods that do not make a difference, that will neither worsen nor improve your PMS. These are the Neutral Foods, and they are approximately equal in calcium and magnesium. They are best avoided if you can choose a food from the *Foods High in Magnesium* List. However, they are much better than the foods on the *Foods to Avoid* List. The foods on the *Neutral Foods* list have magnesium to calcium ratios between 1.0 and 2.0. Remember, the closer the foods you choose are to 2.0 the better the food is for you especially during the week to two weeks of your PMS phase. They are most valuable for women with very severe or very touchy PMS, where the neutral foods can either add to or decrease control over your PMS symptoms.

Table 9

FOODS WHICH ARE BASICALLY NEUTRAL

FOODS WITH HIGH MG/CA RATIO	MG	CA	MG/CA
FRUITS			
Applesauce, unsweetened, ½ cup	4	4	1.00
Apricot, dried, 10 halves	16	16	1.00
Dates, dried, 10	27	29	1.00
Pear, canned, water pack, 1 cup	9	9	1.00
Raspberries, Black, raw, 2/3 cup	30	30	1.00
Cantaloupe, 1 cup pieces	17	17	1.00
Jackfruit, raw, 3.5 oz	34	37	1.00
Kiwi, raw, 1 medium	20	23	1.15
Peach, fresh, 1 medium	5	6	1.20
Peach. canned, water pack 1 cup	15	18	1.20
Persimmon, Japanese, raw, 1 cup pieces	13	15	1.20
Lychees, dried, 3.5 oz	33	42	1.30
Watermelon, raw, 1 cup pieces	13	17	1.30
Melon balls (cantaloupe/honeydew), frozen, 1 cup	17	24	1.40
Tamarind, raw, 1 cup	89	110	1.24
Breadfruit, raw, 1 medium	17	24	1.40
Acerola, raw, 1 cup	12	18	1.50
Carissa, raw, 1 medium	2	3	1.50
Peach, dried, 10 halves	37	54	1.50
Prickly pear, raw, 1 medium	58	88	1.50
Casaba melon, raw, 1 cup, pieces	9	14	1.60
Nectarine, raw, 1 medium	6	11	1.80
Pineapple, raw, 1 cup, pieces	11	21	1.90
Carambola, raw, 1 medium	6	12	2.00

FOODS WITH HIGH MG/CA RATIO	MG	CA	MG/CA
Lychees, raw, 10	5	10	2.00
Plum, raw, 1 medium	2	4	2.00

FRUIT & VEGETABLE JUICES

	MG	CA	MG/CA
Coconut water	58	60	1.00
Orange, fresh, 8 fl. oz.	27	27	1.00
Vegetable Cocktail, 6 fl. oz.	20	20	1.00
Acerola, 8 fl. oz.	24	29	1.20
Prune, canned, 8 fl. oz.	30	36	1.20
Tomato, fresh, 6 fl. oz.	16	22	1.25
Orange, canned, 8 fl. oz.	21	27	1.30
Grapefruit, canned, 8 fl. oz.	18	26	1.30
Grapefruit, fresh, 8 fl. oz.	22	30	1.36

VEGETABLES

	MG	CA	MG/CA
Artichoke, Jerusalem, cooked, 1 medium	47	47	1.00
Chick peas (garbanzo beans), cooked, 1 cup	80	78	1.00
Chive, 1 Tablespoon	2	2	1.00
Brussels sprouts, frozen, ½ cup	19	19	1.00
Mixed vegetables, frozen, ½ cup	22	20	1.00
Tofu, raw, ½ cup	130	127	1.00
Pigeon pea, cooked, 1 cup	72	77	1.10
Soybean, dried, ½ cup	226	265	1.20
Squash, summer, raw, ½ cup	13	15	1.20
White beans, dried, 1 cup	144	170	1.20
Pinto beans cooked, 1 cup	82	95	1.20
Yellow beans, cooked, 1 cup	110	131	1.20
Pink beans, cooked, 1 cup	88	110	1.25
Eggplant, broiled, ½ cup	12	16	1.30
Yams, baked, ½ cup cubed	9	12	1.30
Green peas, fresh or cooked, ½ cup	22	31	1.40
Cow Peas (Blackeyed), cooked, 1 cup	48	66	1.40
Kidney red beans, cooked	50	80	1.40
Poi, cooked, ½ cup	19	29	1.50
Red beans, dried, ½ cup	110	163	1.50
Swiss chard, ½ cup chopped	51	76	1.50
Zucchini, raw, ½ cup sliced	19	29	1.50
Mung beans sprouted, raw, ½ cup	7	11	1.60
Zucchini, cooked, ½ cup sliced	12	19	1.60
Taro, cooked, ½ cup sliced	12	20	1.66

FOODS WITH HIGH MG/CA RATIO	MG	CA	MG/CA
Succotash, canned or frozen, ½ cup	14	24	1.70
Tomato, raw or cooked, 1 tomato	8	14	1.75
Adzuki beans, cooked, 1 cup	63	120	1.90
Lentils, boiled, 1 cup	71	37	1.90
Lima beans, baby, cooked, 1 cup	52	97	1.90
GRAINS, BREADS, PASTAS & CRACKERS			
Pumpernickel Bread, toasted, 1 slice	23	22	1.00
Rice, White, 1 cup	24	28	1.20
Soy Bean, low fat, ½ cup	165	202	1.20
Soy Bean, defatted, ½ cup	297	373	1.25
Whole Wheat Bread, 1 slice	18	23	1.30
French Rolls, Enriched, 1 roll	8	12	1.50
Noodles, Enriched, cooked, 1 cup	16	28	1.75
NUTS & SEEDS (All 1 Ounce servings)			
Almonds, dry roasted	84	84	1.00
Pistachio nuts, dried (47 nuts)	38	45	1.20
Chestnuts, Chinese, raw	27	41	1.50
Hazelnuts, dried/roasted	55	84	1.50
Macadamia Nuts, dried	20	33	1.70
Walnuts, English	27	48	1.80
Sunflower Seeds, dry roasted	20	37	1.85

Table 10

MEATS, POULTRY, FISH, DRINKS AND BEVERAGES

Meat is generally an important part of the American diet. While you can certainly create an excellent anti-PMS diet without any meats in it, most women want at least some meat, poultry or fish on a daily basis. What is important here is that certain cuts of meats, poultry or fish are much higher in magnesium and therefore if you suffer from severe PMS, or brittle difficult to control PMS you will want to know which cuts of meat, poultry or fish to choose.

Meats

Beef averages between a 2 to 2.5 ratio depending on the cut. The flank area tends to run 4.0; ground beef, 2.4 to 3.0; top round, 5.2 and round tip 5.4. T-bone steaks are 4.1.

Poultry

Chicken tends to be in the area of 2 to 1 ratio Mg/Ca depending on the specific parts. White meats tend to be higher in magnesium while dark meats are lower. Duck ranges from 1.5 to 1.8. Turkey averages 2.5 to 1 Mg/Ca. Smoked turkey is higher in magnesium but smoked meats often contain sugar so they may not be a good choice for sensitive women. We suggest staying away from luncheon meats because, with the exception of turkey breast meats, they are generally higher in calcium. All ratios depend on mode of cooking. Roasting meats tends to help retain higher ratios when compared to frying meats.

Most combination vegetable dishes and soups with or without meats or poultry are considerably higher in calcium than magnesium.

Drinks and Beverages

Since water, unless it is distilled, is generally high in calcium, most drinks will also be higher in calcium. Of course, drinks made with dairy products, yogurt, milk, such as malts, milk shakes and smoothies will be high in calcium as well.

We recommend not worrying about the Ca/Mg ratio of your drinks and we suggest that you just use water and other fluids (except those made with dairy products) as much as you want and need as they are essential to your overall health. We generally recommend that every woman drink at least 8 to 10 eight-ounce glasses of water or other fluids each day. While we suggest you do not drink caffeinated drinks (i.e., coffee and teas, etc.), you can drink decaffeinated coffee in moderation (as it still has some caffeine) and caffeine free herbal teas as much as you desire.

Please read labels on soft drinks to avoid caffeinated products and of course avoid all products with chocolate whether caffeine is listed or not. Most foods and drinks which include chocolate *do not list the caffeine within it.*

WHAT ABOUT A VEGETARIAN APPROACH?

The vegetarian approach is generally a major lifestyle change. It is best used by women who have specific reasons, 1) they have severe or very problematic PMS, 2) PMS with severe or problematic menstrual cramps or pain, 3) family or personal history of coronary artery disease, diabetes or significant obesity, 4) significantly elevated blood cholesterol or triglycerides in women who do not want to take medications, 5) women who either want to be a vegetarian or know that they would feel better eating a vegetarian diet.

As you have read through our dietary program for PMS you may have asked yourself if you either have to be a vegetarian or if you so desire, can you live a vegetarian lifestyle and still eliminate your PMS. The answer to the first question is that you do not have to be a vegetarian but, the answer to number two you can easily eliminate PMS using a strictly low-fat vegetarian dietary approach. This dietary approach, when properly followed, has the very helpful effect of reducing the total amount of circulating estrogens, sometimes to a striking degree. For some women a diet that avoids animal products and keeps vegetable oils to a bare minimum can relieve PMS symptoms very rapidly.

There are several reasons why this diet affects hormones. First of all, reducing the amount of fat in the food you eat reduces the amount of estrogen in your blood. This appears to be true for all fats—animal fats and vegetable oils.

Second, plant products contain a good deal of fiber (roughage) and fiber tends to carry estrogens out of the body. As the liver filters estrogens out from the blood stream, it sends down through the bile duct (a small tube for the gall bladder into the small bowel) into the digestive tract. Once estrogen reaches the digestive system the bowel lining will begin a process of identifying estrogen and taking it back up into the body and returning it to the blood stream. When there is an abundance of fiber in the digestive system from eating lots of grains, beans, vegetables, and fruits, the fiber will soak up the estrogens like a sponge and hold it so that it cannot be reabsorbed. When plant foods are a major part of your diet, you will have the abundance of fiber that is necessary to soak up a very large amount of estrogen. However, if your diet is low in fiber, if you eat a lot of low fiber foods such as yogurt, chicken breasts, eggs, or other animal products, you will not have sufficient fiber to make any meaningful difference. Without adequate fiber, the estrogens in your digestive tract end up being reabsorbed back into your bloodstream and thereby maintain the exact same high estrogen level you are trying so hard to eliminate or at least reduce.

Another advantage of a vegetarian diet is that certain foods, especially those that contain phytoestrogens, soy products for one, are also weak plant estrogens however, they can reduce your natural estrogens' ability to attach to your cells. The result is less estrogen stimulation of your cells. While not directly lowering your estrogen level you are reducing the PMS effect created by your own internal estrogens.

Because of all of this, the vegetarian PMS diet can dramatically reduce problems with menstrual pain, and some ovulatory disturbances, irregular periods and such.

THE VEGETARIAN DIET

The vegetarian diet that has been most helpful in treating PMS women excludes all animal products completely and also reduces vegetable oils to very low levels. In order for this diet to work optimally, it must be followed closely. This means no animal products at all—not even skim milk or eggs. It requires keeping vegetable oils to a bare minimum. Even though olive oil or peanut butter are better than chicken fat or beef fat when it comes to cholesterol levels, the effect on hormones is what we are concerned about here, and all fats—animal fats and vegetable oils—are best reduced as much as is possible as they will cause extra estrogen to be made by your body.

So, in addition to keeping animal products out of the diet, it is also helpful to reduce oily salad dressings, french fries, potato chips, butter, margarine, cooking oils, and the shortening that is in many cookies and pastries. It also appears to be important to make this change for the entire month, not just before your period.

For many women this is a very big change in their diet, however, if you have severe PMS it is a relatively fast way to getting your symptoms under control. Good results will be noticeable in the very first month or two after you have made the appropriate changes. It is also a great way to lose excess weight without counting calories. Some people also note that other problems, such as migraines, are less common with this kind of diet.

Before starting lets deal with a few of the common questions that might come up for you if you were deciding whether or not to make the change to a vegetarian diet. You may worry about some of the following topics:

WILL I GET ENOUGH PROTEIN?

Protein is not a problem on vegetarian diets. All plant foods have plenty of protein. Any normal variety of plant products contains more than enough protein for the body's needs.

WILL I GET ENOUGH VITAMIN B6?

Vitamin B-6 (pyridoxine) has been shown to reduce and eliminate depression, irritability, and other PMS symptoms. Vitamin B6 has long been known to be used in the body to protect nerves and as part of the process of making neurotransmitters, the chemicals that conduct our nerve messages. B-vitamins play an important role in controlling estrogens, by increasing their removal from the blood stream by the liver. If your diet is low in B-vitamins, the amount of estrogen in the blood will likely rise.

The healthiest B-6 sources are whole-grains, beans, bananas, and nuts. Refined grains lose much of their B-6 along with their fiber. People eating the typical European and North American diet, are more likely to be deficient in vitamin B-6, because of their high protein intake from the meats, dairy products, and eggs they ingest. These women may require extra B-6.

Studies using B-6 supplements generally use doses in the range of 50 to200 milligrams per day. B6 in dosages over 100 mg per day should be used under the guidance of a physician as higher dosage should be avoided as it can cause nerve problems. B-6 supplements generally take one to three months or more to work.

WILL I GET ENOUGH, OR TOO MUCH CALCIUM?

While there is some evidence which suggests that improving calcium intake can help reduce both PMS and menstrual pain. Generally, it has been our experience that a high calcium intake can be a problem for the women who suffer from PMS-A, anxiety symptoms. Most other women may notice some positive effect with a high calcium diet. Most people tend to believe that increasing calcium intake means that you will have to eat more high calcium food, especially dairy products, or take calcium supplements. However, it may be more important to reduce the amount of calcium your body is losing minute by minute. It is now recognized that animal proteins increase the loss of calcium by increasing the amount of calcium your kidneys have to remove from your blood and excrete in your urine. When people avoid animal proteins, their calcium losses are cut to less than half of what they had been while eating meats.

There are many vegetables, see the Foods to Avoid List, Table 8, and notice those foods that contain high levels of calcium. Calcium is found in a great abundance in green leafy vegetables and beans. You will also find that fortified orange juice is a very rich source of calcium. A plant-based diet will actually reduce the amount of calcium that is lost each day through your kidneys. Hence it will not only provide adequate amounts of calcium but also reduce calcium loss from your body. Also, simple, inexpensive, a calcium carbonate supplements have been shown to reduce PMS symptoms.

Calcium losses can be further reduced by avoiding excess salt in your diet, by limiting caffeine intake to no more than two cups of coffee per day, avoiding tobacco, performing a regular daily exercise program, and making sure that you get sufficient vitamin D, either from regular exposure sun or from a multiple vitamin source. So do not worry about whether you will get enough calcium or not, you can control it and if you eat a basically healthy diet, you will be getting plenty of calcium.

WILL I GET ENOUGH IRON?

Iron in take and balance can actually be better on pure vegetarian diet. Iron is found in abundance in leafy green vegetables and legumes (beans, peas, and lentils) which are both rich in iron and increase your ability to increase your absorption of iron if your body needs more iron, and reduce absorption when your body already has plenty of iron. Avoiding dairy products also helps as they contain virtually no iron and can actually inhibit the absorption of iron into your body. If you already are anemic or worry about becoming anemia, then you should talk with your doctor about taking a good Iron supplement to supplement your needs.

30 Days To No More PMS

WILL I GET ENOUGH VITAMIN B12?

Vitamin B12 is essential for healthy nerves and healthy blood. Vegetarian sources, such as fortified soymilk or cereals do provide vitamin B12, however, since most other vegetarian foods are actually low in vitamin B12 we recommend taking supplement containing vitamin B12. Many authorities believe that this only necessary, to take B12 supplements, if you have been on a pure vegetarian diet for more than three years or started during childhood, while pregnant, or breast feeding, we suggest that you begin vitamin B12 supplementation within the first few months of beginning a vegetarian diet, mainly to make sure that you are getting complete nutrition.

WILL I GET ENOUGH MANGANESE AND ZINC?

Manganese is associated with reduced moodiness and menstrual pain. Manganese along with zinc (See Appendix F) are both essential for healthy sugar metabolism, hence stabilization of blood sugar and indirectly estrogen levels. Your diet should contain adequate amounts of manganese which can be done using a strict vegetarian diet.

WILL I BE GETTING SUFFICIENT ESSENTIAL FATTY ACIDS?

Different kinds of fats act differently in your body. Animal fats contain a great deal of saturated fat, which is the kind of fat that is solid at room temperature, while vegetable oils contain more unsaturated fats, which are liquids. But there are actually many more subtle differences between different kinds of fats.

All fats can directly and indirectly influence the production of prostaglandins in your body. These natural chemicals are involved in inflammation, pain, muscle contractions, blood vessel constriction, and blood clotting. Prostaglandins are suspected of playing a role in PMS, menstrual pain, migraines, and gastrointestinal pains, particularly since many of the pain-killing medicines that are commonly used to treat menstrual pain simply by inhibiting the effects of prostaglandins.

Omega-3 fatty acids tend to help reduce PMS and well as other menstrual symptoms. By adding extra omega-3-rich oils, such as flax oil or fish oils, to your diet you can counteract the "bad" fats in meats and dairy products. Unfortunately, this strategy tends to increase the amount of fat in the diet, which can be risky from several health standpoints and can in some cases worsen PMS. So it is important to watch the total fasts in your diet. On the other hand, a diet high in leafy green vegetables and legumes (beans, peas, and lentils) along with eliminating meats and dairy products can result in a healthier new rebalancing of your diet that still favors omega-3s but reduces the total amount of calcium to allow reduction of your PMS symptoms.

REDUCING THE OFFENDER FOODS

Whether you follow a strict vegetarian diet with elimination of animal products or not the key yo success and elimination of PMS symptoms are still two fold 1) get plenty of magnesium and vitamin B6 on a daily basis, and this can be done by using the Foods To Be Eaten List as we have described above, and 2) elimination or substantial reduction of all processed and refined foods with special emphasis on reducing the daily intake of refined sugars and caffeine.

THE ROLE OF REFINED SUGAR

Refined or simple sugars can contribute to irritability and depressed mood. Researchers have found that refined sugar increases the amount of the brain neurotransmitters which control moods. In our experience, individuals are affected by refined sugar very differently than with normal fruit and plant sugars. For some women, especially just before a period is due, a bar of chocolate or any other sugary food—even orange juice— can cause a dramatic increase in irritability, while other people have a much more mild reaction.

While sugary foods, especially chocolate, are often craved during the premenstrual period, it is well worth avoiding them as an experiment to observe the differences in how you feel.

Foods that are rich in complex carbohydrates and fiber, such as whole wheat bread, brown rice, oatmeal, vegetables, and beans, do not seem to cause moodiness, and higher protein foods, such as beans or tofu, tend to help block the effect of sugar on moods.

ROLE OF CAFFEINE

Caffeine aggravates PMS, and the more caffeine you consume—in coffee, tea, colas, or chocolate—the worse your PMS is likely to get. Caffeine should be avoided as much as is possible.

HOW DO WE CALCULATE A MG/CA RATIO?

The magnesium and calcium contents of the foods listed below are in milligrams (mg.) per 100 grams (100 grams is equal to approximately 3.5 ounces) of the food. Occasionally, the units of measure may differ and, if so, the exact unit of measure will be stated.

The magnesium/calcium ratios are calculated by dividing the number of milligrams of magnesium by the milligrams of calcium. The number produced indicates the relative proportion of magnesium to calcium. The larger this number, the greater the amount of magnesium in the food. On the contrary, the smaller this number is, the less magnesium and the greater the amount of calcium in the food.

For example:

Sweet corn contains 48 mg. of magnesium and 3 mg. of calcium per 100 grams.

Therefore:

48 mg. of magnesium divided by 3 mg. of calcium ($48 \div 3$) = 16.0; or 16 times more magnesium than calcium.

The Mg/Ca ratio can be stated as either 16 mg. of magnesium to each 1 mg. of calcium, or as 16 to 1

We abbreviate this as a 16:1 food

Now no matter how much corn you eat there will always be 16 times more magnesium than calcium.

Let's try one more example of determining the Mg/Ca ratio of a food. For this food let's determine the Mg/Ca ratio of a baked potato with its skin left on (as the skin is an excellent source of magnesium). The whole baked potato contains 54 mg. of magnesium and 22 mg. of calcium, therefore: $55 \div 20 = 2.5$ (rounded off).

For each of the foods in the three lists, the Mg/Ca number represents the ratio of magnesium to calcium. When we state a figure such as 16.0 for corn or 2.5 for potatoes, as in the examples, we mean that it is a sixteen to one (16:1) or a two and eight-tenths to one (2.8:1) ratio of magnesium to calcium.

PICKING YOUR FOODS – THE THREE COMMANDMENTS OF ADVANCED PMS DIET

Rule Number One: **Eat only foods you like.**
Rule Number Two: **Learn to like the foods that are most healthful for you.**
Rule Number Three: **Forget rule one until you are symptom free.**

In order to make yourself symptom free it is valuable to be somewhat adventurous. You may need to try foods you previously had biases against. We hope this won't be a problem, but if you look at the food lists and tell yourself that you are not interested, or don't like the majority of foods on the Desired Foods List, the dietary program will not work for you unless you are willing to change your eating habits, what you choose to eat, take risks and become much more adventurous.

We want to make sure that you have a large variety of foods to pick from so that you can eat whatever you like, whenever you like, in order to help eliminate your symptoms. In addition to the food lists, we will give you a number of hints that will help you to get all of the nutrients you need to enjoy life, be well and be symptom free.

As we said above, take your time and learn to recognize the foods that are good for you as well as those which can worsen your symptoms. As we suggested earlier, you will find it extremely helpful in the beginning to make up your own lists of Desired Foods and Foods to Avoid which you can carry in your purse for immediate use. This will enable you to have a list of *your* favorite high magnesium foods as well as a list of your most problematic high calcium foods available whenever or wherever you need them. It is likely that you will soon learn which foods work best for you. In a short while you may be ready to set your list aside and just go from what you know works and what doesn't work for you.

To help you understand how to pick food, we would like to run through a number of examples with you. Quite often, we have women tell us that even though they are eating "the way they are *supposed* to eat," they continue to have problems. This is usually because they are not using the lists, haven't thought out their meals and they are not eating the way they think they are.

The following example will quickly demonstrate how easy it is to eat in a way which causes PMS and how easy it is to eat your way out of your PMS

EXAMPLE #1

How about a nice, green salad, with lots of carrots, cucumbers, some beautiful ripe tomatoes, some delicious low-fat mozzarella cheese and to top it off, a low-fat Italian dressing. A nice lunch, wouldn't you say? Low calorie, low fat, plenty of fiber. Sounds good, doesn't it? But us it going to decrease or increase your PMS symptoms?

Let's look at its makeup in relation to PMS; especially its calcium and magnesium content:

	Calcium	Magnesium	Mg/Ca Ratio
Lettuce, Romaine, 3½ ounces	68 mg.	11 mg.	0.2
Carrot, 1 medium, raw	19 mg.	11 mg.	0.6
Cucumber, ½ cup sliced	7 mg.	6 mg.	0.9
Mozzarella cheese, part skim	207 mg.	7 mg.	0.03
Tomato, ½ raw	4 mg.	7 mg.	1.8
Italian dressing, 2 tbsp.	4 mg.	2 mg.	0.5

Now let's add it all up:

The salad as it is above contains:	**480 mg.**	**44 mg.**	**0.14**

...and

How about some Rye Krisp crackers?	2 mg.	8 mg.	4.0

This salad may look good and even taste good, but it will not help you to eliminate your PMS. In fact it may make it worse.

"Well," you say, "what if we eliminate the cheese, after all cheese is dairy and dairy is higher in calcium, isn't it?" You are exactly right so lets see what happens when we do this.

	Calcium	Magnesium	Mg/Ca Ratio
The salad with cheese contains	309 mg.	44 mg.	0.14
Mozzarella cheese, part skim	-207 mg.	-7 mg.	0.03
The salad without the cheese	**102 mg.**	**37 mg.**	**0.4**

Well, that helped, a little, but the mozzarella also has some magnesium so it didn't help really all that much, did it? We did increase the Mg/Ca ratio from 0.14 to 0.4 a definite improvement, but not one that is going to help us very much.

How about if we leave the cheese out but add 2 nice rye krisp crackers to the lunch?

	Calcium	Magnesium	Mg/Ca Ratio
The salad without the cheese contains:	102 mg.	37 mg.	0.4
2 Rye krisp crackers	24 mg.	68 mg	2.8
Total Lunch: Salad and Rye Krisp	**126 mg.**	**105 mg.**	**0.8**

Well, this helps a little more, but we are still not anywhere near 2.0 or more where we will be getting help for your PMS.

If we analyze this carefully, we'll find that this meal has 1.2 times as much calcium as magnesium. (The Mg/Ca ratio is 0.8, we want to go to 2.0 at least hence we still need to more than double the total amount of magnesium without changing the amount of calcium..this is not going to happen easily.) This meal would not help you treat your PMS. Now can you see why it is so easy to eat yourself into PMS. Notice that this meal is not a bad meal. Almost anyone would tell you that this is an extremely healthy way of eating, except if you are trying to avoid PMS.

EXAMPLE #2

Now let's add some more high magnesium food to this meal. We will add more foods from the Desired Foods List. Let's look at the Desired Foods List and see if you can find some foods which are relatively high in magnesium (and of course, vitamin B6). There are a number of foods which we can add into our lunch and can be eaten along with the salad which will immediately increase the amount of magnesium.

Let's trade the mozzarella for something else, for example, avocado, cashews, peanut butter, baked potato or corn on the cob.

	Calcium	Magnesium	Mg/Ca Ratio
Salad without cheese	102 mg.	37 mg.	0.4
Avocado California, 1 medium	19 mg.	70 mg.	3.7
Total for Lunch & Mid Afternoon Snack	**121 mg.**	**107 mg.**	**0.88**

Notice now that the calcium has increased only slightly but the magnesium has more than doubled. The amount of calcium is now just a fraction above 1.13 times as much magnesium. The Mg/Ca ratio is now 0.88. This meal is moving more toward neutral rather than PMS provoking.

EXAMPLE #3

In the process of increasing magnesium and making this meal a better anti-PMS meal, let's add a side of black beans. Sound good? Watch and see how you can eat yourself out of PMS and love it.

	Calcium	Magnesium	Mg/Ca Ratio
Salad with avocado & rye krisp	**121 mg.**	**107 mg.**	**0.88**
With a side of black beans	47 mg.	121 mg.	2.6
Total for Lunch	**168 mg.**	**228 mg.**	**1.4**

137

We have now reversed the Mg/Ca ratio and have more magnesium than calcium. While we still do not have a great deal of magnesium in this meal, we are far ahead of what we started within the beginning. This one meal isn't going to solve your PMS problem, but at this point it won't make your PMS worse. Now in the next set of examples let's see how we can get you to a 2 to 1 or better ratio through the remainder of the meals and snacks of the day.

EXAMPLE #4

If you were to have a mid-afternoon snack of 1 ounce of dry roasted cashews, you will further increase the magnesium total for the whole day.

	Calcium	Magnesium	Mg/Ca Ratio
Lunch	168 mg.	228 mg.	1.4
Cashews (1 oz., dry roasted), a snack	13 mg.	74 mg.	5.7
Total Lunch plus Snack	**181 mg.**	**302 mg.**	**1.7**

The numbers are now getting better and better. We are now at 302 mg. of magnesium and your Mg/Ca ratio is now at 1.7. This is mid-neutral, not worsening and possibly lessening your PMS symptoms.

EXAMPLE #5

Now let's look at dinner:

	Calcium	Magnesium	Mg/Ca Ratio
Baked potato, one medium	22 mg.	54 mg.	2.5
Turkey, white meat, 3 oz.	6 mg.	15 mg.	2.5
Peas and carrots, 1/4 cup, steamed	8 mg.	26 mg.	3.3
Total Lunch	36 mg.	95 mg.	2.6
Add to Lunch and Snack above	181 mg.	302 mg.	1.7
Total Lunch & Dinner	**217 mg.**	**397 mg.**	**1.8**

Now you're at a total of 397 mg. of magnesium and a Mg/CA ratio of 1.8. We have moved forward but we're still not at the 2:1 ratio. However, we have forgotten all about breakfast today. So let's go back and look at what you could have eaten for breakfast.

EXAMPLE #6

If, at breakfast you had eaten a bowl of oatmeal fortified with some rice bran, your outlook might well be entirely different at this point.

	Calcium	Magnesium	Mg/Ca Ratio
Oatmeal, Quick, ¾ cup	15 mg.	42 mg.	2.8
½ Tbsp. Rice Bran	10 mg.	160 mg.	16.0
Add Ex. 3, 4 and 5 above	217 mg.	397 mg.	1.8
Total All Meals for the Day	**242 mg.**	**599 mg.**	**2.5**

Now, the total amount of magnesium for the day is 599 mg. and the Mg/Ca ratio, is at 2.5 magnesium to 1 calcium. Your diet for this day would not only reduce your symptoms but even help eliminate them.

EXAMPLE #7

We still want you to have a morning snack, for that is extremely important in order to maintain an even blood sugar level, giving you energy and managing your PMS:

For your morning snack let's have:

	Calcium	Magnesium	Mg/Ca Ratio
Banana, 1 medium	7 mg.	33 mg.	4.7
Apple juice, 8 oz., frozen or fresh	14 mg.	12 mg.	0.9
Add Ex. 3-6 above	242 mg.	599 mg.	2.5
Total All Meals & Snacks for the Day	**263 mg.**	**644 mg.**	**2.5**

Your total magnesium is now 644 mg and while Mg/Ca Ratio is still only 2.5 which is well within the upper range of helping to resolve PMS symptoms, we have added more sugar to your system to fight hypoglycemia and to maintain a relatively even blood sugar.

While the morning or afternoon snacks don't always substantially change the Mg/Ca ratio, they do help maintain adequate daily blood sugar, as well as helping to maintain a constant flow of magnesium into the body.

USING VITAMIN-MINERAL SUPPLEMENTS

One quick way to get your Mg/Ca ratio up into a range that would diminish your PMS symptoms is to use vitamin-mineral supplements. There are a number of good products on the market. If this does not meet your needs, we suggest that you look for a vitamin-mineral combination that has a Mg/Ca Ratio of at least 2 to 1 or, preferably, 3.2 to 1 ratio. That is, the product you buy should have somewhere between 200 to 400 mg. of magnesium and no more than 125 to 200 mg. of calcium in a day's supply. Conveniently, many companies package their products in the form of five or six tablets for a day's supply. Each tablet contains both magnesium and calcium. This packaging allows you to divide your supplements up during the day. To insure that you have a relatively even flow of magnesium into your body throughout the day, you should take one or two per meal and one with each snack.

The Right Supplement Will Help You to Control Your PMS Much More Rapidly and Give You an Excellent Jump Start Toward Complete Elimination of All of Your PMS Symptoms.

Any supplement chosen should be a multiple vitamin-mineral complex which contains at least a minimum of the RDA amounts of Zinc, Chromium, Selenium, vitamin E and a full complement of the B vitamins including at least 100 to 300 mg. of vitamin B6. Amounts considerably greater than RDA levels are often used. These are called *Mega-vitamin* dosages and are quite common. While in working with PMS we are primarily interested in magnesium and calcium and vitamin B6, for good health and well-being any supplement you purchase should be well-rounded and provide sufficient vitamins and minerals to eliminate any other vitamin-mineral deficiency that might be present.

Some women choose to maintain their magnesium levels by taking supplements and eating whatever they choose regardless of the total amounts of magnesium and calcium. Women who have mild PMS can often do this. However, the more severe the PMS is initially the start the harder it is to maintain the proper Mg/Ca balance and get good results. While the supplement raises magnesium levels rapidly, a diet high in calcium can just as easily reverse its value.

Vitamin Toxicity

Vitamin A: 100,000 IU per day for any period of time, possibly grater than one to two months, can lead to toxic symptoms.

Vitamin D: 100,000 IU has been noted as top level above which there generally is not benefit. Toxicity may be in the range of 300,000 IU per day for more than 1 to 3 months.

Vitamin E: Therapeutic doses of vitamin V range from 300 to 2,000 IU per day. Toxicity occurs in only two groups of people 1) high blood pressure patients' 2) chronic rheumatic heart disease patients.

Vitamin B6: Toxicity has been reported with doses in excess of 200 mg per day for several months.

Table 11

The best plan is to always do it right. Make a good portion of your diet high-magnesium/B6 foods and eventually you can eat what you want without having to rely on a supplement. Supplements can then be used to support your diet, to supplement you on "bad" days and to support you when you "cheat."

In the remainder of this chapter, we will give you more information about the foods that will help you as well as the foods that have created and perpetuated your symptoms. Our intention is to make you familiar with both the good and not so good foods. We believe that when you have a full understanding of what must be done and why you must do it, you will have no conflict in changing your eating habits.

DESIRED FOODS – FOODS HIGH IN MAGNESIUM

As we have repeatedly stated, one of the most important aspects of the nutritional-dietary approach in treating PMS is the elimination of excess calcium especially for the PMS-A women, where calcium makes PMS symptoms worse, and the supplementation of magnesium.

We now know that relief of PMS symptoms can best be accomplished by:

1. Picking foods especially high in magnesium and relatively low in calcium.
2. Eliminating (a) those foods which are high in sugars (especially, refined sugars), fats, dairy

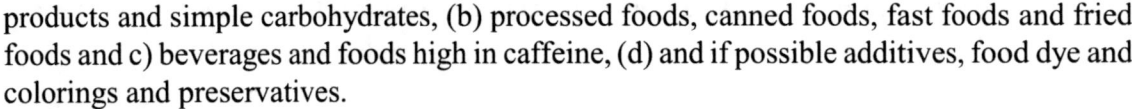

products and simple carbohydrates, (b) processed foods, canned foods, fast foods and fried foods and c) beverages and foods high in caffeine, (d) and if possible additives, food dye and colorings and preservatives.

3. Taking vitamin-mineral supplements (when necessary).

For some women those with particularly moderate to severe PMS all of these steps are necessary. In order to help you get the best results with the least amount of supplements, we are providing you with two main lists of foods: *Desired Foods – Foods High in Magnesium* and *Foods to Avoid – Foods High in Calcium*. These two lists can be used by you to help pick foods that are high in magnesium and low in calcium. As you learn how to use these lists, you will not only reduce your symptoms but also reduce the amount of supplements your body needs to control and then eliminate your PMS.

Since *calcium is necessary for you*, we do not want you to eliminate it entirely. In fact, you would not be able to do this even if you tried very hard. Calcium is so common that it is impossible to really reduce it in your diet. If you were to add up all of the calcium and magnesium in your diet, you will soon see that there is really a great deal more calcium than magnesium.

We understand this. We want you to understand this. But we know that it is important to get your daily intake of magnesium up into the 400 to 600 mg. range for a while. To do this we have devised this program to help you eliminate your symptoms and plan high-magnesium meals and snacks. These lists will help you accomplish your goal.

On the Foods High in Magnesium List we have placed the high magnesium foods in decreasing order, from foods with the highest Mg/Ca ratio down to those with the lowest Mg/Ca ratio. The absolute amounts of calcium and magnesium are also important and must be watched if symptoms remain a problem.

> **Once You Learn How to Eat Correctly,
> You Can Essentially Eat Anything
> and Everything You Want and
> Still Be Able to Remain
> Symptom Free.**

FOOD LISTS TO SUPPORT ELIMINATING PMS

Throughout the course of our book you will find a series of food lists which will present a series twenty different types of foods. Each of these food lists are each divided into three parts: (1) Foods

To Be (entirely) Avoided, and (2) foods which can be considered relatively neutral, Neutral Foods List, and 3) Desired Foods List, which are foods that are good for you. Each of these groups are determined by the individual foods Calcium to Magnesium Ratio. Foods which are greater than 2.0 Mg/Ca ratio are High Magnesium Foods, Neutral Foods are foods with Mg/Ca ratios between 2.0 and 1.0 and finally, Foods to Be Avoided have Mg/Ca ratio which is less than 1.0.

FOODS TO AVOID - FOODS HIGH IN CALCIUM

Foods to Avoid, are generally best avoided entirely, if possible, during the critical period of the menstrual cycle, that, is the two weeks prior to the onset of the menstrual period, the time when PMS symptoms are often at their worst. These foods will tend to stimulate PMS and **make** your symptoms worse. They are high in calcium and relatively low in magnesium. These foods have ratios less than 1.0. **Remember:** The smaller the ratio number the more calcium (also the less magnesium).

The foods in the second list can be considered Neutral Foods. That is, they are approximately equal in calcium and magnesium. They are best avoided if you can choose a food from the Foods High in Magnesium list. However, they are much better than the foods on the Foods to Avoid list. The foods on the Neutral Foods list have magnesium to calcium ratios between 1.0 and 2.0.

Section III

The 30-Day To No More PMS Program

WEEK 1: DAYS 1-7

1. The first step of the 30-Day program is to read our book from cover to cover and become aware of your PMS symptoms and what PMS is.

2. Go to the Forms Section in the back of the book and print a copy of our **Premenstrual Evaluation Questionnaire (PEQ)** and then complete this brief questionnaire and then score it to determine if you have PMS and how severe it may be.

3. Go to the Forms Section in the back of the book and print a copy of your **Personal Management Diary, *Daily Symptoms Record*.** Read the directions and then start immediately using this form to record your symptoms on a daily basis.

4. Go to the Forms Section in the back of the book and print a copy of the *My 10 Most Favorite Foods* list. Next read the instructions and then fill this form out to the best of your ability.

5. Review the Most Desired Foods and Foods to Avoid Lists. Compare your choices on *My 10 Most Favorites Foods* list with these two lists and determine if you consume sufficient magnesium in your diet.

6. Bases on your PEQ Score (Step 2 above) determine whether you have mild, moderate or severe PMS symptoms.

    a. If you have mild or mild moderate PMS start on our Basic PMS Diet in Chapter 5, Section I.
    b. If you have moderate or severe PMS symptoms then go to Chapter 5, Section II, reread and understand the Advanced PMS Dietary Program. Between the Basic Dietary Program and working to increase your magnesium-to-calcium ratio in the foods you eat, start your new anti-PMS diet.
    c. Decide whether or not you will need to use supplements.

7. If you believe that you need supplements then shop to find the best formula available to you. If you wish you can go to our website and order our Metamorphosis Women's Formula I, which is designed to support you and our PMS diet.

8. Begin a comfortable exercise program, join a gym or get out and walk, dance more or bicycle, read the PMS and Exercise Section and create a daily exercise program. Start slow and easy.

WEEKS 2 THROUGH 4

1. Work on adding more high magnesium food to your diet and eliminating refined and processed food, refined sugars.

2. Read labels on everything your pick up and certainly on everything you buy.

3. Continue to increase and add to your daily exercise program. Remember to start and go slowly. Add steadily, as you can tolerate, to your exercise program. Remember you do not want to over do it in the beginning, so do a little less and never too much. Do not injure your self, tire yourself out to exhaustion or make it so hard you hate doing it.

4. Continue to improve and modify your anti-PMS diet by reducing refined and processed foods, and by continually adding more and more high magnesium foods. Watch your symptoms and if your PMS-A symptoms are not going away or worsening, then reduce calcium foods until your symptoms are finally under control.

5. If you are not taking vitamin-mineral supplements than make sure that you pick sufficient foods

high in vitamin B6 on a daily basis. See the Food High In Vitamin B6 List in Appendix C.

MONTH 2 AND SUCCEEDING WEEKS AND MONTHS

1. If you started with mild to mild-moderate PMS symptoms you should be almost completely symptom free during month two.

2. If you started with moderate to severe PMS and you have followed the program as outlined you should already have noted significant improvement in your PMS symptoms. If you have not noted improvement then you are still doing something wrong.....DO NOT GIVE UP...instead reevaluate what you are doing and tighten up your diet. If you are not taking supplements then start as soon as possible.

3. Continue to add high magnesium foods, adjust calcium foods intake and reduce refined and processed foods until you are entirely symptom free. Maintain yourself being symptom free for six months and then you can switch entirely to the Basic PMS Diet as your daily Maintenance Diet.

4. If you cheat significantly, then either add more magnesium and vitamin B6 to your diet for a while or use your vitamin-mineral supplements to cover you for a while until you can go back to the Basic PMS Diet alone.

Since there is no luck involved, we will wish you only good healthy eating........

SUMMARY – HOW TO USE THE 30-DAY TO NO MORE PMS PROGRAM FOOD LISTS

In the High Magnesium Food List magnesium is listed first, then the calcium value for each food, finally the Mg/Ca ratio. Foods are generally listed in descending order of highest magnesium foods first down to lowest magnesium and hence Mg/Ca Ratio value last. In the Foods To Avoid list we have placed the calcium values first, next magnesium and finally Mg/Ca Ratio's. Foods on this list are ordered from the least desirable to the most desirable Mg/Ca Ratio's. The entries steadily increase toward those foods which are highest in their Mg/Ca ratio. This is only to allow you to visualize the relative amounts of calcium to magnesium. As the numbers increase, the relative amounts of magnesium increases and the foods become less of a problem.

The reader should take note as to how many more high calcium foods there are than high magnesium foods. It may become much more obvious as to why PMS is such a common problem in our society. We usually suggest that each woman make a list of the 10 most common foods (you can use the 10 Most Common Foods Form in forms Section at the back of the book) she eats and note how many of them are likely to be foods which are high in calcium rather than magnesium. If you do this for yourself, we believe that you will certainly be able to see why you have PMS.

The values for magnesium and calcium on these lists come from several sources. Where considerable disagreement occurs between sources both values are listed. The values given are not averaged in any way. They are representative values and indicate the approximate levels of magnesium and calcium for a specific food. Foods can vary widely in vitamin and mineral content depending on where they were grown, how early they were picked and the methods of preparation.

CHAPTER 6

THE FULL SCOPE OF PMS

PMS is one of those areas of medicine in which the medical community has taken little interest. Perhaps it's because it exists entirely in women and is not considered life threatening by the medical establishment, or possibly this occurs because men *expect* women to be illogical and erratic.

PMS is down-played today not only by the general public but by OB-Gyn's and other medical practitioners. Often, women who suffer from PMS are not taken seriously. They are frequently perceived of as faking symptoms or treated as if it is all in their head. To change the attitude of the professional and lay communities toward PMS, it will take publications, like our 30-Days to No More PMS program, to seriously address the problem. It is possible that PMS is discounted because somewhere deep in our *knowing* we realize that this syndrome is a simple problem with a relatively simple solution.

It is clear, however, that this simple problem with a relatively simple solution creates complex and even occasionally life threatening problems for the unfortunate women who are unaware that there is a simple solution. In the introductory chapters of our 30-Days to No More PMS program we discussed at some length the many physical and emotional symptoms of PMS. We acknowledged that symptoms can become so severe, so painful and so seemingly hopeless that it can cause some women to try and often to succeed at suicide. We have also discussed the wide range of effects PMS has on self-image, well-being and quality of life. We have looked at the mood swings, bloating, swelling, palpitations, difficulty in sleeping and the characteristic depression that is commonly seen with PMS.

So far however, we have merely discussed the symptoms of PMS. To completely understand PMS we must also examine a number of the medical and social problems which are in one way or another related to PMS. Of the conditions we are about to address only one has been directly connected to PMS. For the others a direct "causal" relationship cannot be claimed at this point. In some cases, however, the interrelationships are quite striking. It is not our purpose to make a case to prove a cause and effect correlation but rather to educate the readers of our 30-Days to No More PMS program and to demonstrate the relevant parallels. These conditions, which are common in women with PMS, occur more often than would be statistically reasonable. It would seem that it would take very little work on the part of a observant physician to notice this.

We would like to make it clear that we do not necessarily believe that any or all of these conditions are caused by PMS but rather that there is some type of relationship between them that must be investigated. If the treatment and resolution of PMS would help eliminate or slow down any of these other processes, then this must be considered an extremely important step. Lastly, if there is a causative association, then controlling PMS would be essential in the prevention and treatment of these conditions.

Although we know that PMS appears to be associated with elevated estrogen levels, the exact degree of elevation and the role of estrogen-progesterone ratio, its overall effect on any one woman's body and organs are not easy to determine. In this Chapter we will in the first section presented some brief information about the medical problems related to PMS and in the second part of this chapter we will look at a number of the more important social, psychological and spiritual problems related to PMS. The following common gynecologic problems we are about to present are frequently found to coexist with PMS. Many of them are already known to be caused by high estrogen states. Once again while we cannot be sure that they are caused by PMS, we know that they are indeed linked with it in some way.

SECTION I

MEDICAL PROBLEMS ASSOCIATED WITH PMS

ENDOMETRIOSIS

A condition in which cells, identical to those which line the uterus, appear to implant upon and within many of the pelvic and abdominal organs. These cells form island-like structures which act exactly like the cells of the lining of the uterus. That is, they are hormonally responsive. They change with the cyclic hormonal changes which are affected by the release of estrogen and progesterone. As estrogen levels rise, these cells are stimulated to grow. In a sense, they are preparing themselves for the implantation of a fertilized egg. They do this even though they are outside of the uterus and cannot possibly be part of the reproductive process. Eventually, when the body recognizes that a pregnancy has not occurred, these cells breakdown and *bleed* into the tissue upon which the endometrial cells have become implanted.

Endometriosis characteristically is associated with discomfort or pain starting one or more days prior to menstruation and ending shortly after the onset of menstruation. Once we started observing our patients with endometriosis we realized that virtually every woman we treated also had PMS. Interestingly enough however, not all women who had PMS had endometriosis. Over the past years, there have been few, if any, articles published in the research literature that relate these two high estrogen conditions together.

Whenever we work with a woman who has endometriosis we make sure to treat her PMS as well as her endometriosis. We recommend that every woman with endometriosis be treated with the same anti-PMS diet which we have presented within our 30-Days to No More PMS program. Dietary treatment is not to be used instead of the medical treatment recommended by your doctor but, rather, as an adjunct to it and along with it.

FIBROCYSTIC DISEASE OF THE BREASTS

Fibrous and glandular changes in the breasts are fairly common problems that affect women all over the world. This condition has long been associated with elevated estrogen. Recently there have been many articles that suggest that a diet high in caffeine and high in saturated fats may predispose to these benign tumors. Recent treatment programs have suggested reducing caffeine and saturated fats and adding high doses of vitamin B6 and vitamin E and other vitamins. We encourage women with fibrocystic breast disease to participate in the anti-PMS diet to help lower circulating estrogens. Once again, not all women with fibrocystic disease of the breasts also have PMS. This fact might suggest that there may be more than one cause for this condition. Most of the women we have treated with our dietary program seem to improve quite rapidly and significantly. The mega-dose vitamin-mineral supplements, which was discussed in an earlier chapter, are often very helpful in treating this condition.

MENSTRUAL IRREGULARITIES

Irregular bleeding, intramenstrual spotting, and prolonged menstrual bleeding are often caused by an elevated or impaired estrogen-progesterone ratio. Often women who have irregular uterine bleeding also have PMS on occasion irregular bleeding may be their only symptom. The anti-PMS diet is often helpful in reversing the estrogen-progesterone imbalance and stopping the irregular bleeding. The medical treatment for this group often depends on the pattern of bleeding and the age of the patient. Life-style factors such as use of oral contraceptives, degree of stress, amount of activity, other medications, etc. must also be taken into consideration. When cancer or uterine polyps are suspected, a Dilatation and Curettage (D&C) is often necessary for diagnosis and even treatment. In young women with PMS symptoms where cancer is not a high risk, the anti-PMS diet may be tried before more radical hormonal or surgical treatments. Once again the diet should not substitute for appropriate medical diagnosis and treatment. It should act only as an adjunct to it.

INFERTILITY

Infertility, a difficulty in getting pregnant, can be related to either the male partner or to the female partner and, in some cases, to both. Once again, while not all infertile women have PMS, many do. Since PMS is an elevated estrogen condition, it is possible that the underlying cause of their PMS may also play a role in potentiating their infertility. In this case, either the nutritional deficiency or

149

the hormonal imbalance it causes might well be the culprit. If infertility is in any way directly related to an estrogen-progesterone imbalance, or the nutritional imbalance which causes it, then these women are excellent candidates for this good, healthy diet we suggest for PMS women.

PROBLEMS DURING PREGNANCY

PMS women may be at higher risk for early miscarriage, threatened miscarriage, migraine headaches associated with pregnancy, preeclampsia and toxemia of pregnancy. Many of these problems appear to be greatly minimized when the pregnant woman is placed on our good, healthy diet. It is likely that PMS women who get pregnant have a higher than average risk for the conditions we just described. Generally, the relationship between PMS and problem pregnancies has been missed by most OB-Gyn's. Unfortunately, many women still suffer and are subsequently placed at risk when it is now, for the most part, unnecessary.

Women who enter into pregnancy and do not realize that they have PMS, may have an increased likelihood of developing preeclampsia or toxemia. PMS women also have an increased likelihood of developing postpartum blues or a full-syndrome postpartum depression. As we have suggested earlier, PMS may not manifest itself until a woman becomes pregnant. Since PMS is associated with multiple pregnancies are associated with PMS, we suggest that all women who desire to get pregnant, who are already pregnant or who have had multiple pregnancies start immediately on our anti-PMS diet program. During pregnancy we are less concerned about the need to reduce calcium levels (as pregnant women need more calcium). We are however, more concerned about the use of processed foods, simple carbohydrates and overcooked, fried and less than fresh foods. These foods have diminished nutritional value. Since the pregnant woman has an increased need to provide nutrition for herself and her baby, we are adamant about having pregnant women strive to eat only fresh, high quality, healthy, natural foods and drinks. This is essential to our diet and this is why our diet program is perfect for the pregnant woman.

FIBROID TUMORS

Fibroid tumors of the uterus occur quite frequently. The origin of fibroid tumors has long been connected to irregular and elevated estrogen levels. Most commonly associated with menopause and the years just before it (perimenopause), fibroid tumors are less frequently identified with PMS. Whether this is because PMS is often entirely missed is hard to say. In our experience, we have found that many women with fibroid tumors suffer from PMS or had been suffering from PMS until symptoms of the perimenopause appeared to take over. Occasionally, like women who are pushed out of balance by pregnancy, women are thrown out of hormonal balance by the transition and the onset of menopause.

Most physicians are aware that these muscle tumors of the uterus are stimulated by elevated estrogen. Hence, a diet that could normalize irregular swings of estrogen could be beneficial. The fact is, we have seen this many times. When the fibroids are small the anti-PMS diet may well be most helpful in decreasing excess circulating estrogen whether the woman has overt PMS or not. When the fibroids are large they may require surgical removal. Once again the PMS diet is helpful in the pre-op phase to protect against the stresses of surgery and subsequent development or worsening of PMS after surgery.

MENOPAUSAL SYNDROME

The symptoms of the menopause are directly related to irregular, often widely fluctuating, swings of estrogen caused by the gradual failure of the woman's reproductive system. While many organ systems lose their sensitivity to estrogen, others are over-stimulated, especially the uterus, the breast, the brain and other hormonal organs. In this process, a set of characteristic signs and symptoms develop which we call *symptoms of menopause*. These symptoms are often not substantially different from those found in PMS. On the other hand, sometimes the symptom patterns are sufficiently different enough to immediately demonstrate that we are dealing with two entirely different problems. Clearly, however, there is overlap where those women with PMS transform into women with PMS and perimenopausal symptoms. Eventually they may simply become a woman with menopausal symptoms only.

Once again, since both syndromes relate to a certain malfunction of estrogen, the anti-PMS diet, a good, healthy diet, could certainly have efficacy as part of the treatment regime for menopause. It could correct PMS problems and help stabilize estrogen metabolism until the menopause is complete. It is possible, but not yet proven, that in the untreated perimenopausal women the irregular swings of estrogen may directly or indirectly lead to such conditions as endometrial and breast cancers.

The problem of osteoporosis associated with menopause and post menopause alone warrant being on this diet. The high levels of magnesium in the blood stream force calcium into the bones. Besides minimizing osteoporosis, the reduction of circulating calcium reduces the chances of osteoarthritis, bone spurs, gall stone and kidney stone formation. The increased level of magnesium which forces calcium into the bone also reduces the potential for hardening of the arteries. When calcium levels are needed to be increased, if there are signs of osteoporosis, such as decreased bone density, the total amount of magnesium in the diet should then be increased to its highest tolerable levels.

GENITAL CANCER

Uterine (endometrial) cancer and some forms of breast cancer are also known to be related to elevated levels of estrogen and impaired estrogen-progesterone ratios. The anti-PMS diet may help to control the estrogen level and therefore might have some efficacy in the prevention or treatment of these genital cancers. Once again, it should not be used as a substitute for competent medical treatment, but rather, as an adjunct to it.

Although the conditions listed above have not been definitely proven to be related to PMS, in many cases there appears an unexplained relationship between them. It may be that some of these conditions will ultimately be found to be directly associated with PMS in the future, while others will be found to have no association with PMS. Until scientific proof one way or the other is established, women can only benefit by the nutritional-dietary approach and appropriate follow-ups for the other conditions.

POSTPARTUM DEPRESSION

There are at least two types of postpartum depression. One type appears to be directly related to PMS-D group, while the other predominantly a psychiatric type seems unrelated. The PMS version differs significantly form the normal postpartum "blues" that occurs with the let down created from the normal drop in hormonal levels immediately after birth. The depth of the depression caused by PMS after delivery is often more profound and deeper then the more usual postpartum "blues." Woman with PMS postpartum depression apparently cannot tolerate the hormonal disruption to their nervous system easily. PMS postpartum depression needs to be treated immediately and taken seriously as in their depressed state they can take actions which may ultimately bring harm upon themselves or their infants. That is why the treatment of the PMS-D woman in the postpartum period first requires replacement of the missing hormones, that is she must be given moderate to high doses of estrogen along with some progesterone in order to prevent vaginal bleeding.

Women with existing PMS-D symptoms demonstrate a significantly greater risk of postpartum depression. In one study PMS women had a 43% chance of postpartum depression while postpartum depression only occurred 12% of the time in women without PMS. Other factors when associated with PMS that seemed to be related were, past use birth control pill and PMS postpartum depression was 91.6% more likely to occur as verse to 45.9% increased likelihood in non-birth control pill users with PMS, alcohol use with PMS occurred 39.5% more often than in women with little or no alcohol use, and illicit drugs use in PMS women, 48.4% more likely to occur than in non-drug users with PMS. In this study there was a clear association between these factors and PMS. They should be identified in women with PMS during the initial visit, and their role in the creation or worsening PMS and potential postpartum depression should be watched and evaluated.

Characteristically, the woman who will ultimately suffer from PMS-related postpartum depression will also more likely suffer only mild to moderate nausea during her first trimester and then will experience a period of general well-being, and no further nausea during the next two trimesters. When this occurs the obstetrician should always watch for potential PMS related postpartum depression after delivery. It seems that women who suffer from more severe nausea and vomiting are less likely to suffer from severe PMDD.

This combination of events, appears to relate directly to depression that is hormonally related and associated with the occurrence of PMS either before or after the pregnancy. In some situations, as with preeclampsia and toxemia, there may be no signs of PMS prior to the pregnancy. It is likely that these women are marginally nourished prior to their pregnancy and that their hormonal/nutritional systems becomes unbalanced some time during the course of the pregnancy. It is also possible that their estrogen-progesterone ratio had remained relatively normal even in the face of significant nutritional and hormonal imbalance. Then with the strain of pregnancy they were ultimately pushed too far so that ultimately their PMS symptoms appeared during or after their post partum period.

During our many years of working with this dietary program, we have noted that few pregnant women who have been on a really good, healthy diet have ended up having major complications during pregnancy or postpartum depression afterward. On a number of occasions women who were referred to us with postpartum depression responded faster to treatment when this dietary program was part of the overall treatment regime. We clearly believe that all women with postpartum depression, even postpartum blues (the milder form) should be under appropriate medical and psychological supervision, either by a psychiatrist or an Ob-Gyn and a psychologist but they all should also be eating a good anti-PMS diet as well. As usual the extent and intensity of this diet should depend on the severity of their individual symptoms.

It should be remembered that approximately 5% of these women will manifest the symptoms from the depression group of PMS. Treatment of these women should include a small to moderate amount of estrogen hormone. This is especially true if they were previously treated with natural progesterone and their PMS symptoms worsened.

DEPRESSION

Depression is one of the more common symptoms of PMS. PMS depression must be differentiated from non-PMS depression this is best dome by determining if the depression symptoms occur on a cyclic basis related to the menstrual cycle in the week to two weeks prior to the onset of menstruation. If depressions symptoms are cyclic then it relates to PMS, if not then the depression is not related to PMS. Severe depression related to PMS is PMDD, see below.

PREMENSTRUAL DYSPHORIC DISORDER (PMDD)

This condition is a severe depressive syndrome related to PMS, it has been discussed in great detail in Chapter 1, starting on page 13. We will not be adding anything to this prior discussion at this time.

SECTION II

SOCIAL AND SPIRITUAL PROBLEMS RELATED TO PMS

PMS AND ITS EFFECT ON THE FAMILY

There are many ways PMS can and does affect the family. The most obvious effects are related to the changes in your behavior and the symptoms that you may suffer from. In an earlier section of this book we have listed the many symptoms of PMS, some are common and others are much less common, even rare. If you have any of these symptoms, especially those that affect you emotionally or physically, then it is likely that they will now or in the future, to some degree or another, be obvious to others, and most especially to family members, friends or even co workers. If they affect you, then it is most likely that they will also have some effect on one or all your family.

Some of the most common symptoms that effect the family are those associated with significant (that is, obvious to others consciously or unconsciously) depression, anger, acting out, mood swings or irritability. Often women are unable to recognize the full extent of the effect of their PMS on themselves and therefore will miss its effects on their family. PMS women have been brought into us by their husbands (or a parent) with instructions, as one husband told us, "Fix her before I have to file divorce."

PMS very often has a significant negative affect on children. Often children, especially young children, have no idea as to what is normal and abnormal, and what is caused by PMS versus a crazy, irrational mother, sister or even grandmother. When a mother acts out from PMS her children will often accept her acting out either as being totally normal, the way ALL mother act, or they may think that their mother is "crazy," or at least that something is wrong with her. As one young girl told us, "Sometimes my mother is just not my mother. I always wonder where my real mother goes, until she comes back again." Children may even believe that *all* women are supposed to act this way, that PMS is normal behavior.

Young girls may even believe that when they grow up, this is the way they are supposed to act or that "being PMS," is normal. Often because they do not know any different, children may emulate their mother and exhibit PMS behavior. Young boys may from an early age think of their mother, and hence all women, as erratic, emotional and unstable. Because of the acting out, erratic behavior, broken promises, sudden fits of anger and rage that PMS women are subject to, their children may soon believe that their mother (and possibly all women) is not to be trusted or relied upon.

We wonder, in the need, how many divorces are caused by PMS, how many children have given up on their mothers and how stereotypes are created so easily from a condition, PMS, which is fully and completely treatable.

PMS AND THE ADOLESCENT TEENAGE GIRL

It is also extremely important, when we discuss PMS and its effect on the family, to discuss the relationship between PMS and teenage girls. While statistics tell us that PMS occurs more commonly in women during their mid to late twenties, what is overlooked is that this is often when PMS peaks, and that in fact, PMS generally begins much earlier often in early teens.

PMS symptoms can begin almost anytime after the onset of the menstrual cycle. Most commonly symptoms do not reach the point where they are enough of a problem to require medical attention until somewhere between 25 and 35 years of age. The exception to this would be during the period of adolescence. Adolescent PMS often presents a number of special problems which require a brief discussion of their own. While everything we have said about PMS applies to adolescent girls there are some unique differences.

During adolescents two factors encourage the problem of PMS. 1) Adolescents is a time of significant fluctuation of female hormones, estrogen and progesterone. 2) Some adolescents have estrogen levels that become extremely high, ovulation may occur some months and not during other months. In the months that it does occur there may be significant possibility of an imbalance of estrogen-progesterone ratio, on top of this, since the exact right estrogen-progesterone ratio may not yet even have been established for the young woman, PMS symptoms may well not occur in some months, be severe in others , mild in still others and swing wildly from month to month ,making it look more like the young girl is out of control rather than PMS.

MORE ON THE ROLE OF DIET IN ADOLESCENT PMS

During the formative years of childhood children, often develop specific likes and dislikes related to food. During the teen years many teens have poor diets, living on hamburgers, fries, malts, shakes, candy, power bars, junk foods and developing severe nutritional deficiencies. Once the child has established her food preference *list* the die is cast as to her later development of PMS. If the young girl selects a diet which is similar to our anti-PMS diet it is unlikely that she will have PMS problems. However, if her dietary likes and dislikes run more along the line of a diet which stimulates PMS then she is likely to develop PMS some time in the future.

Because PMS is usually associated with adult women, teenage girls can have some or all of the symptoms their mother's may have or have had, or they may have an entirely different pattern. Too often teenage girl are ill prepared to deal with the negative feeling created by their PMS. Because of this there are a number of "symptoms" that are particularly problematic in teenage girls. Since

PMS can begin anytime after onset of menstruation, physicians and parents should begin watching for signs of PMS from this point on. Especially if there is already an existing family history of PMS in mother, sisters, grandmothers or maternal aunts. It is not at all unusual by 16 years of age. The youngest girl we have diagnosed with PMS, of whom we are aware, was a 14-year-old. The youngest girl with PMS whom we have personally seen in our practice was a 16.

PMS is often missed in teenage girls because *no one is looking for it.* PMS symptoms in girls below the age of 19 often go unrecognized and are frequently missed. Generally, teenage girls do not see gynecologists regularly and if their mothers and fathers are not very knowledgeable about PMS, they will not consider it no matter what symptoms, issues or problems their daughter is having. If the mother has significant PMS she may miss her daughter's symptoms because of being so involved with her own problems. Also, the symptoms of PMS in teenagers is often very different from PMS in the adult women. Many people believe that the teenage years are *supposed* to be erratic and turbulent, but all too often the girls with extreme behavior problems may be experiencing symptoms of PMS.

In younger girls the symptoms of PMS tend to be somewhat different from those of adult women. Symptoms in adolescent girls tend to be much more erratic in nature and are less likely to have a recognizable pattern. In young girls erratic behavior is more likely to be accepted as normal. Mood swings and irritability appear to be present all month long and the worsening prior to menstruation is often missed or just written off as teenage tantrums. This usually occurs because these young girls generally have no idea as to what is normal or abnormal. The girls rely on their parents, especially the mother, to let them know if something is wrong. Parents often rely on the doctor to tell them if something is wrong with their child. Since the mother and her doctor are usually not well educated about PMS, early PMS symptoms are frequently misdiagnosed.

Since PMS in adolescent girls is most commonly manifested as behavior problems, all mothers should be aware of the types of problems which might indicate PMS. The most frequent symptom is cyclic depression and next, is some form of acting out. One particularly disturbing behavior problem is sexually acting out (sometimes to the extent of nymphomania), others are alcoholism, drug use and addiction, running away from home, tantrums, feeling unloved, and occasionally suicidal behavior.

Dr. Dalton studied PMS in adolescent girls and found that they were more likely to be in trouble at school as well as with their parents or with the law. They had a high incidence of such problems as petty theft, shoplifting, lying, setting fires, vandalism, child abuse (the adolescent's abuse of a brother or sister or her own child), increased absenteeism from school and poor grades. They may exhibit an unwillingness to act in accordance with their parent's or with the requirements of other authority figure.

Most important of all, just as with adult women, these symptoms tend to be cyclic in nature. While erratic behavior may occur irregularly or even daily during the month, it is especially a problem in the week to two weeks prior to the onset of menstruation and seems to improve or disappear suddenly with or shortly after the onset of menstruation. Since some adolescents girls will not ovulate every month, symptoms may not occur in those months when they do not ovulate, making PMS much more difficult to diagnose.

These symptoms do not necessarily imply that the child is "bad." Many girls outgrow these behaviors. These are simply the same types of irrational, mood swing, depressive types of symptoms which adult women experience. It seems, however, that in the adolescent these symptoms are more often markedly exaggerated. The main problem is that these behaviors can significantly affect the adolescent girl for the rest of her life. An unwanted pregnancy, a police record, alcoholism or drug addiction, a record of being a child abuser or arsonist can seriously alter the direction of this child's life.

The greatest majority of young women do not get into severe problems. But for many, impaired habits, the loss of self-esteem and a lowered self-image can create problems that are often extremely difficult to overcome, if indeed they can ever be resolved.

First, there is an alarmingly high rate of suicide among teenage girls with PMS. PMS often causes severe depression and some of these girls are unable to deal with their dark moods and fears effectively. They may not feel that their problems are in any way solvable and that there is no one there for them to turn to. They may experience their symptoms as being something inside of them, that they are just "bad seeds," or more rightly that something is wrong with them, but because they are unable to explain what is happening, they are embarrassed or no one is listening or caring, they often go untreated. Some girls begin to feel that suicide is the only way out. This is the primary reason that any teenage girl who is depressed, moody, talking about suicide, performing suicidal-like behaviors, or acting suicidally *must* be evaluated and PMS should always be considered as a primary or contributing factor.

Suicidal behavior has two meanings here. One is the standard meaning of attempting or actually committing suicide. The other is that they may be doing suicidal things such as using large amounts of alcohol, drugs, driving erratically, unprotected, indiscriminate sex, bad relationships, running away, alienation from the parents and other friends. Often these are seen as emotional problems, but they may actually be caused by PMS or emotional problems may exist and they are potentiated by the girls PMS. Those girls with PMS need to be treated for their PMS, whether they need psychological counseling or even psychiatric medication, will be determined by which is their primary problem. If psychiatric issues are primary, then these should be treated first and PMS that is also occurring should be treated next. If PMS is the primary problem then the PMS should be treated and the girls watched as to how they respond to the treatment of their PMS.

A second problem is nymphomania or sexually acting out. Estrogen is a stimulant and is well noted by the anxiety type of PMS, When estrogen is elevated the sex drive is increased. This is a built in mechanism to ensure the survival of our species. When the teen aged girl has PMS she has elevated estrogen levels. Too often, however, the teenage girl is ill prepared to deal with the negative feeling created by her sexually acting out. Her budding sexuality and her need for love may overwhelm her

and her inability to control her emotions may lead her to sexually acting out. She maybe driven by these negative forces into nymphomania, multiple partners and indiscriminate sex. This behavior may occur only during PMS portions of the cycle or it may occur all month long. It is not unusual for the teenager to lose her self-respect and feel as if she has a tarnished self-image and ultimately become so severely damaged that she feels driven into running away or even engaging in prostitution. Early pregnancy and marriage may also be secondary effects of untreated PMS.

A third problem is teenage obesity. Here once again as with her adult counterpart, cravings, low self-esteem, low ego strength, mood swings and depression may come together in the form of excessive appetite, overeating, binging and weight gain. This weight gain separates her from her, "ideal - perfect self-image" which worsens her depression, exaggerates her mood swings and makes her more unhappy, withdrawn and feeling unloved. This drives her cravings and psychological need for food which leads to binging and more weight gain. It is a vicious cycle and no matter how hard she tries she cannot seem to break it, with the exception of possibly falling into self-starvation, purging and other eating disorders. Identifying if PMS is the cause or contributes to such behavior is essential. If PMS is found, it should be treated. The Basic PMS diet can easily be modified to help teenage PMS girls simultaneously lose weight and reverse her PMS.

A fourth problem is alcohol, alcoholism and drug abuse. We referred to this above. Many teenage girls, who would otherwise be trustworthy and reliable, end up as alcoholics or drug addicts because they are trying to eliminate their PMS symptoms (deal with mood swings, depression, anger, etc.) Alcohol addiction is quite common in PMS women. Alcohol, being basically pure sugar, will temporarily relive the cravings and sugar blues that PMS women are subject too. Unfortunately, it only relieves them for a short while. Hence after the first drink the symptoms will return again and because of the high sugar content of the alcohol the symptoms will now be worse then they where before the first drink. Now she needs another drink to take away these symptoms and a deadly cycle is instituted. Soon she is addicted to the alcohol as well as relieving her PMS symptoms. The reliance on alcohol along with a lowered self image can easily lead to many girls to alcoholism.

The same thing happens with drug addiction except her the woman stops eating and begins to starve herself this too triggers PMS. She may in fact, be using drugs to lower her appetite either to lose weight or because she somewhere inside of herself recognize the relationship of PMS to what she is eating. Hence, it has a slightly different mechanism than alcoholism in teenage PMS drug abuser, but in the end the result is the same the drugs are needed to cover up the negative feeling and PMS symptoms.

A host of other problems can result. These stem from the same factors, inability to control themselves, PMS symptoms and low self-esteem and low ego strength. They include behavior problems, poor grades, cutting school, pick the wrong friends, sexual acting out, shoplifting, fighting with siblings, hostility toward parents and the establishment, and much more.

ADVICE TO THE PARENT WITH A PMS TEENAGER

First and foremost learn everything you can about PMS. If you have PMS there is a good chance that your mother did before you and that your female children will after you. Since a major problem in the creation of PMS is diet, it is extremely important that you work with your children (all of them, boys and girls) to learn how and what to eat. You now have all the information you need to do this so it is ultimately up to you and your desire to protect your children as to whether you go this extra mile. Boys at the adolescent ages also experience hormonal extremes because of their maturation process. This can be helped by giving the boy's body what it needs, in a dietary sense, to support is new hormonal changes. It is just as essential to limit or eliminate the offender foods in your male children as it is in your female children.

Determine whether your teenager is eating the typical PMS diet, foods high simple carbohydrates, processed foods and foods with high sugar content, caffeinated foods and beverages, as well as food dyes, colorings and additives, all of which have long been identified with behavior problems, hyperactivity and acting out and PMS.

Start working with your children as early as you can. The earlier the better. If you get to them before they have established their own likes and dislikes it will be much easier to help them. Do not force them to eat any food that is on our desired food list. Often when children are forced they will rebel. Just offer them fresh, wholesome, good foods as often as you can and demonstrate that these foods are (and we hope they are) part of your favorite way of eating as well.

You will get much better results with love and *enrollment*, that is, getting them to do what you want because they see you enjoying it and they want to emulate your likes and good feelings. Most important of all try to keep them away from the offender foods, especially foods high in sugar, simple carbohydrates, packaged foods, artificially coloring or flavoring and caffeine.

Often parents use sweets to bribe their children into doing what the parent wants, as a treat for good behavior or as a pick me up when the child is unhappy, depressed or upset. The underlying message becomes sweets and sugary foods will make you feel better. It is no surprise that when life doesn't go exactly the way your child wants, she will open a quart of ice cream or down two or three chocolate bars. Rather than sweets, use hugs and special time together. Use healthy foods like fruits or vegetables, such as carrots, or sugar free, whole grain breads or cookies.

When your daughter reaches the age of the menarche (the time of onset of menstruation, usually ages 10 to 14) sit down and tell her about menstruation. Let her know about the hormonal changes and how her diet can affect her. Mothers are often fearful to breach this topic. Year after year we see women who were terrified when they first started to menstruate, having no idea what was happening to them. They often fear that something must be radically wrong with them because no one prepared them for it.

Tell your child about your problems with PMS. This is extremely important for several reasons. When children do not know that PMS exists or what it is they often believe that their mother's behavior is either the normal way women are supposed to act or that there is something wrong with her.

PMS women have frequently confided in us that while they were growing up they thought their mothers were crazy because of their erratic behavior. Only when they personally were confronted with PMS and began to recognize the same pattern of symptoms in themselves and found out about PMS were they finally able to begin to understand that their mother's behavior was due not to insanity but rather to PMS. Some of these women also confided that they put off seeking help for their symptoms because they thought it was hereditary. Since mother had it, they believed that they were destined to suffer as well.

PMS in adolescents can be prevented only by proper diet and education of parents about the signs and symptoms of PMS in the adolescent female. If you have children, give them a positive sense that PMS is a natural consequence of an inadequate diet and that it can be corrected by a diet which provides appropriate nutrition using good, wholesome foods. Teach your daughters what you have learned and you may give them one of the best gifts ever, quality of life and good health. They may never have to suffer with the extremely severe symptoms you had.

It would generally be an excellent idea for every parent (whether PMS already exists in the family or not) to have their teenage girl evaluated for PMS. This is especially true, if she is acting out or exhibiting *any* of the symptoms or cyclic behavior related to PMS. This can be done as simply as taking her to a medical doctor who is competent in recognizing PMS or even having her complete the *Premenstrual Evaluation Questionnaire* (PEQ).

If your teen age girl is found to have PMS, she should be clearly informed about what PMS is, what causes it and how it should be treated. She should be started on an anti-PMS diet immediately. If she is unwilling to be on a diet (which we believe to be the very best treatment) she may be willing to take special supplements formulated to reverse PMS. If none of these are acceptable, she may prefer medical treatment including progesterone or antidepressants, mood elevators, or even menstrual period suppression.

We believe that the safest and most reliable treatment to eliminate PMS is a proper anti-PMS diet.

CHILD ABUSE AND SEXUAL ABUSE

In an earlier section we discussed the relationship between sexual abuse and PMS and we noted that there was a significantly increased likelihood of prior sexual abuse in PMS women. There is also an increased risk for physical, mental and emotional abuse ans well as child abuse related to PMS.

As the PMS woman is caught up in her PMS crises in the week to two week period before the onset of her menstrual period she suffers from many of the symptoms of PMS. Because of the symptoms she may irritate her partner and he may respond in an abusive way. Also PMS women tend to have lower self esteem, use alcohol, are more likely to spend less time qualifying partners so they often risk not only sexual abuse but also physical, mental and emotional abuse.

The PMS woman is also more likely to abuse her children as they may get on her "nerves" when she is highly irritable, depressed or moody. PMS does not excuse any of this behavior neither on the part of the woman nor her partner. But it is more common and it is also a good reason to recognize that medical attention is needed and should be sought after sooner than later.

SPIRITUAL CONFLICT AND PMS

While we tend to resist the concept of an individual having a spirit in medicine we cannot leave it out when it comes to PMS. The rigors of PMS, the many symptoms, the mood swings, depression, irritability various other symptoms can take the life out of any woman and leave her broken, troubled and confused. When this happens there are two ways out 1) treat the PMS, and 2) connect to your inner faith. PMS can cause a spiritual warp or it can strengthen your spiritual bonds, It is up to you as to which it does. Pick the way that leaves your stronger and healthier.

SECTION III

WHAT IS NEXT?

CAN I TREAT MY PREMENSTRUAL SYNDROME ENTIRELY BY MYSELF?

We have been repeatedly asked this question over the years, the answer is **Yes**. However, this assumes that you will do whatever is necessary and exactly what works. Anyone can treat a condition like PMS. Getting the results desired is, however, another issue. While we could certainly say "Yes" to your ability to treat yourself, we cannot promise results unless you know what you are doing, you do what works and you keep doing it until you get it right.

PMS, while annoying and sometimes incapacitating, is generally neither dangerous nor fatal, in itself, without any of the extreme side affects as we have discussed above. We believe that every woman should be treated, whether her symptoms are mild or severe. It is also true that by the time most women recognize that they have PMS, their symptoms are either very distressing or on their way to becoming so. As you will see in Chapter 4, The Medical Treatments of PMS, symptoms can have severe debilitating and on a very rare occasion even have life threatening consequences. This one of the main reasons why we urge early recognition and treatment. Further, we believe that the dietary changes necessary to eliminate PMS are generally easy to learn, simple to establish and are healthful and nutritious.

Therefore, whether you are treated in a professional setting or you treat yourself, PMS must be treated. Our goal in our 30-Days to No More PMS is to get this message across and help you to get the very best results you can get. Your ability to self-treat through the nutritional-dietary approach depends entirely on your willingness to learn and your ultimate desire to succeed. It is also important to be aware that your ability to get immediate results will depend on the severity of your PMS symptoms. The milder your symptoms, the more likely you can be treated by diet alone without medical support. The more severe your symptoms, the more likely that either vitamin-mineral supplements or some form of medical treatment may be necessary to get you started. The earlier you recognize your symptoms and the more motivated you are, the more likely you are to become symptom free.

In the next part of this chapter we will provide you with a tool which can help you to determine not only whether you have PMS but also its severity. This tool can be used to determine the level of the PMS Program you should start with: 1) diet alone, 2) diet and supplements or 3) diet, supplements and natural progesterone.

USING THE PREMENSTRUAL SYNDROME EVALUATION QUESTIONNAIRE (PEQ)

To help you determine the severity of your PMS symptoms, we have included an evaluation form which we call our *Premenstrual Syndrome Evaluation Questionnaire or PEQ*. Please read the instructions carefully and fully and then complete the PEQ. You can down load a PEQ form our 30DaysToNoMorePMS.com from the Forms Section or complete the PEQ provided in the Personal Forms Section below.

1. Using a scale of 0 to 4, with 0 = No symptoms at all, 1 = A mild level of symptoms, 2 = A moderate level of symptoms, 3 = A severe level of symptoms and 4 = Incapacitating symptoms, grade those PMS symptoms you are experiencing in the week before, during your period and the week after your period.

2. Once you have completed your PEQ add up each of the three of the columns and place the scores at the very bottom in the boxes marked for totals.

3. Now in the far right column place the total of all of the boxes in Column A. Below that place the total of all of the boxes in Column C, now subtract the total form Column C from the total from Column A and put this number in the box marled for Severity of Symptoms below the other two boxes. You have now rated your own PMS symptoms. From this number using the scale below you can determine how mild or severe your PMS is.

Go to the Forms Section in the back of the book for additional printable copies.

GRADING YOUR OWN PMS

Now that you have established your PMS score let's see how you have done. The lower this number is, the better off you are. If you scored below 12, you can consider yourself essentially symptom free, thus you do not have PMS. A total between 12 and 20 means that you are borderline PMS. A total score which is greater than 20 definitely suggests you have PMS. The higher your score is above 20, the more severe your PMS is likely to be.

As a general guide, women who score between 12 and 20 usually can be treated simply using the Basic Dietary Program only. This means increasing magnesium and vitamin B6, reducing dairy products, sugar and other simple carbohydrates and eliminating processed foods and caffeine during the second two weeks of the cycle. This is often sufficient to obtain excellent results. See Chapter 6– Section I Basic PMS Diet.

The closer the score is to 20, the stricter the dietary controls will have to be in order to become symptom-free and to maintain this state on an ongoing basis.

Women who score between 21 and 30 are generally considered to have mild to moderate PMS symptoms. These women will more than likely require considerable attention to their diet using the Advanced PMS Diet, read Chapter 6– Section II along with the use of vitamin-mineral supplementation until the dietary program is well established.

As your score moves closer to 30, it signifies that symptoms are progressing from moderate to severe. This group is likely to require increasingly stricter dietary control to create and maintain a symptom-free state. Strict diet control means increasing high magnesium foods and almost complete elimination of sugar, refined foods, alcohol, caffeine, preservatives and additives and high calcium foods in both dairy and vegetable forms. It will also be necessary to take a daily vitamin supplement as well as to paying strict attention to maintaining a high magnesium diet throughout the entire monthly cycle.

Scores greater than 30 clearly indicate severe PMS. It is extremely likely that these women will need very strict dietary control along with large dosages of supplements. While many of the women in this group can maintain themselves with diet and supplementation alone, some may not be able to do this for quite a while. These women may require treatment with natural progesterone either in the form of suppositories or injections, along with their dietary and supplement regime. It may take several months or before the dietary program is firmly entrenched and working well.

Women who score greater than 35 on the PEQ will generally have very severe PMS symptoms. They frequently require natural progesterone along with strict dietary control and vitamin-mineral supplementation on a continuing basis for several months until they become symptom free and have clearly adapted to the anti-PMS diet.

The PEQ results are to be used simply as a guide to illustrate where you are at the time you score yourself. The results do not predict where you will be in the future.

IF I USE PROGESTERONE, DO I HAVE TO STAY ON IT FOR THE REST OF MY LIFE?

The answer to this question is, No! However, your ability to wean yourself off of natural progesterone will depend on your body's chemistry. With application of a strict dietary program and natural progesterone, most women find that after a short time their symptoms begin to diminish. Their PEQ scores drop and they eventually are able to discontinue use of progesterone to diet and supplements. As the PMS symptoms further improve, supplementary dosages can be reduced and, in many situations, even dietary restrictions can be lifted.

Some women have such narrow metabolic states that they require progesterone or supplements for long periods of time. Finally, a small number of women seem to require one or both indefinitely. However, once they have resolved their initial deficiencies, most women are able to control their symptoms by diet alone.

In virtually all situations, PMS symptoms disappear with the onset of menopause. Occasionally, however, menopausal women who take high doses of estrogen along with relatively low doses of progestogens may develop PMS-like symptoms. When this happens, diet and the adjustment of the dosage of estrogen or even the use of natural progesterone may be necessary. If your symptoms do not go away you are generally either still deficient (not on the program long enough or not getting enough magnesium and vitamin B6) or you are doing something wrong (not eliminating enough of the Offender Foods).

HOW DO I KNOW WHETHER THE TREATMENT IS WORKING?

There is only one way to know whether your PMS dietary program is working for you and that is by the results you are getting. When you are using the optimal combination of the right diet (as we have already outlined) of supplements and/or of natural progesterone, the symptoms will just "go away." Yes, as we have repeatedly stated, it is just that simple. When the vitamin-mineral imbalance is returned to the normal range, your symptoms will seem to magically disappear. This is exactly the way it is with almost every other vitamin or mineral imbalance. If you do not trust yourself use this Daily Symptom Diary (In the Forms Section at the back of the book) and record your symptoms on a daily basis and watch the numbers go down.

WHAT KIND OF PREPARATION IS NECESSARY BEFORE TREATING MY PMS?

You should have a complete physical examination. This examination should include an evaluation of the heart, lungs, blood pressure, liver and kidneys. A pelvic examination should be done to evaluate for cancer (pap smear), uterine size and fibroid tumors, for endometriosis and for ovarian tumors. A thorough breast exam to evaluate for cancer of the breast as well as for fibrocystic disease of the breasts should be part of this examination. Blood tests for anemia, blood cancer (leukemia), diabetes, thyroid, liver and kidney function should also be performed. Hormonal studies are rarely necessary as they are usually too insensitive to pick up the estrogen-progesterone ratio defects. Cholesterol, HDL and LDL fractions, as well as triglycerides, may be helpful in evaluating your cardio-vascular status for prevention of atherosclerosis. This exam and laboratory evaluation is necessary to be absolutely positive that there is no other problem but PMS.

A computerized dietary analysis may be helpful in evaluating your present diet (which got you into PMS) but it is not absolutely necessary. We have already given you all the information you will personally need to determine whether you have PMS and what you are eating to cause it. One can determine calcium and magnesium intake, but probably more important is the evaluation of your intake of sugar (especially hidden and unknown), simple carbohydrates, processed foods, alcohol, caffeine, food and chemical additives and fats in your diet.

Hair analysis, considered controversial in its value, may have a place in comparing dietary intake with the content of magnesium and calcium in the hair. Although still a new field, this can frequently add valuable information in otherwise extremely difficult, resistant or complicated situations.

(This Page Is Purposefully Left Blank For You To Use To Take Notes)

CHAPTER 7

EXERCISE IS ESSENTIAL FOR TREATING PMS

STARTING YOUR EXERCISE PROGRAM

Exercise has long been recognized as having a positive effect in reducing, or in some cases even eliminating, PMS symptoms. Since PMS generally occurs in younger women and because women who have or have had PMS tend to have a higher incidence of menopausal symptoms the belief is that starting a regular exercise program early and making it a priority can also work to the woman's best interest in reducing her risk of osteoporosis later on. For all women a regular exercise program, especially aerobic exercise can help to maintain a healthier heart and healthier respiratory system and lower the risk of cardiovascular disease, stroke and high blood pressure. In the following section we will give you some tools, hints and information which can help you to strengthen your heart and improve the condition of your entire body.

BEGINNING A HEALTH EXERCISE PROGRAM

The first and foremost there are two questions which you must ask yourself. "Do you *really* want to exercise?" and if so, "What effort are you really willing to put into it?" Depending upon the answers you gave you will find out whether or not you are really motivated to create a regular on-going exercise program. The very best form of motivation is exercising for the right reasons: "I deserve to look better." "I deserve to feel better through exercising." "I will have everything I desire, including optimal health and well-being." When coming from the right place creating a regular on-going exercise program is a product of a mandate between you and yourself made for loving and caring reasons, for bettering yourself.

If this is your motivation then you will want to exercise to tone your entire body, to feel better, to look better and to be healthier. To accomplish these goals you will want a safe means of exercising, one where you can start slowly, build up slowly and work at your own speed, and one in which you can get everything you want without injuring yourself. The best form of exercise to start with in order to accomplish these goals is walking.

STARTING TO WALK

When starting an exercise program walking is the easiest, safest and possibly the best form of exercise to start your program. Like any other venture in life, proper preparation can make all of the difference. Once again review why you are doing this and who you are doing it for. Make a firm and committed decision to do it and lastly, to do it for the right reason.

Do not start until you are ready. Purchase a good pair of walking shoes so that you do not hurt your feet or end up being fatigued and uncomfortable. Wear comfortable non-restricting clothes which both protect you from the elements and keep you from over heating.

Begin your walking exercise program simply by getting out and walking. When we say walking we are not talking about strolling where you look in shop windows, that is for a lazy Sunday or shopping Saturday. Not are we talking about running or jogging for they are not walking. Walking should be brisk and rapid. Your arms should either swing freely by your sides or be used to almost "pump" yourself on, that is, they should be bent at the elbows and briskly moving the forward and backward timed with each step, helping you propel yourself forward.

In the very beginning make your walks short, just to the place where you feel good and feel as if you have done enough for this particular day. DO NOT over do it. If you do too much you will be exhausted and you will not want to do it again. Go until you reach the place where you are feeling exhilarated and stop as a winner, feeling good, ready and willing to repeat your experience again tomorrow or the next day, because it feels so good. Do not worry about how far you go or how long you are walking. Listen to music or a book on tape if you desire. Walk only where and when you can assure, as best as is possible, your safety. Never walk alone at night nor in any isolated area. Bring a friend who also wants to walk. Walk in a place where there are people. Remember your safety is paramount.

MAKING IT AN EXERCISE PROGRAM

Now you are walking, but this is not yet, necessarily an exercise program. To create an exercise program you will want to do it regularly and make it an integral part of your life. As you do this you can now gradually increase the amount of time and distance you walk. To do this simply and safely each day go just a bit further or walk a bit longer than the day before until you are doing a solid 20 -30 minutes a day five or more days a week or 30-45 minutes 3 days a week. As you become proficient and feel you need an additional challenge then there are several things you can do: 1) Add 1 pound ankle weights on each foot. (But do this only when you are ready, and do this slowly). 2) Add 1 pound weights around each arm. Gradually build these weights up to 2 pounds all the way up to 5 pounds on your legs and 1 to 3 pound on your writs. 3) Once you have mastered this than read The Intermediate Walkers, later on in this section.

HINTS FOR THE INEXPERIENCED WALKER

If you are ready to start walking here are a number of helpful hints to make it easier, safer and more productive.

4. If you are not a conditioned athlete then you will want to start out slowly for the first few weeks.
5. You should walk only distances that you are comfortable walking.
6. Walk in a safe area so that you feel secure and protected. If possible, walk with a friend or even several friends, although this is not essential.
7. Do not walk with a dog unless it is well trained and disciplined. Too often dogs will want to stop at every bush or tree to mark territory. This slows your walk and limits your goal. If this happens a lot you are really not getting the exercise you need or desire.
8. If you desire to listen to music consider the following: pick music that is up beat and will help you maintain a pace you can manage without tiring rapidly. The music or whatever you listen to should not impair your ability to hear vehicles coming toward you, children playing in your path or an intruder. The music should not take away your attention to the path, where you are walking nor impair your safety.
9. When you first start, walk only until you feel energized and enlivened, then stop. If you exhaust yourself, you are less likely to want to walk again the next day.
10. Do not push yourself to the point of fatigue or exhaustion as this will destroy your willingness to exercise regularly.
11. Go slow, take your time in building speed and endurance, wait until walking is a regular pattern and you feel ready to move yourself up to the next level.
12. Once you have created a habit of exercising and you feel good about exercising you can start pushing yourself more and more and working toward complete physical fitness. It is most important however to first create the habit of exercising.
13. If you are new to exercising, exercise only every other day or every third day. As you get more and more fit and into exercising, you can progress it to every day, 15 to 30 minutes or more.
14. Use your upper body as much as your lower body. Make your walking a full body experience. This not only improves the toning of the upper body and makes the exercise more cardiovascular in nature but increases significantly the total number of calories burned which can go a long way to helping you control your weight, if this is an issue.
15. If you have back or limb problems consider a reclining bicycle or swimming. Never do anything that can hurt you, cause pain or exhaustion. Build slowly and steadily.
16. If you chose to walk in-doors either find a walking track such as a YMCA or other health club or use a treadmill.
17. If you have a home treadmill all of the above still apply, do not overdo it, gradually build up the difficulty, time, speed and resistence on the treadmill. Do not try to do too much too fast. Be safe, do not hurt yourself.

HOW WALKING WORKS TO HELP YOU

Walking requires energy. Your muscles get their energy from *fat* stored within the muscles. This fat is turned into called *glycogen*. Glycogen is made in the liver from this fat and is stored in the muscle for its eventual use. Exercise improves utilization and production of insulin and stabilized the hormonal system all of which ultimately impact your estrogen production and its removal from your body. During the process of exercising your body will release *endorphins*, and these neurochemicals will make you *feel* better. You will then have more energy and you will feel better, which will reduce or counteract the negative symptoms of PMS.

When you start to exercise, glycogen is burned as fuel. If you walk long enough or hard enough you will eventually burn up all of the glycogen and your muscles will move into *an anaerobic metabolism*, that is, they will start to produce lactic acid.

While you are walking, you do not directly burn fat, however but once you stop walking and your stored glycogen has been burned up, it then must be replaced and this can only happen through what you eat and by the liver drawing fat from fat tissues. If you are on a limited caloric intake then the food you take in will be used basically for feeding your brain and the energy for your exercise will then be drawn from your fat stores which will have to be drawn on to replace the glycogen used up while exercising. Hence, you burn body fat, lose fat, feel better, reduce your weight, reduce or eliminate your PMS symptoms all at the same time when you exercise regularly.

Since the upper and lower extremities represent a very significant portion of the body's muscular tissue the amount of fat burned can be quite substantial when you develop your upper body. Another interesting fact is that after you have walked for a while the body actually returns more glycogen to the muscles than they had started with in the beginning. It does this to prepare for your needs to walk (or run) again in the near future. It does this to protect you and prepare you for potential danger. Walking, therefore, burns up more fat than the energy used during the process of walking alone.

If you now continue to walk on a daily basis (at least once or possibly even twice a day) more and more fat will be burned, more endorphins will be released, and your extraneous body fat will decrease (assuming you are also on a reasonable caloric intake for your height and weight and level of exercise). Since fat stores extra estrogen, and this extra estrogen that contributes toward your PMS symptoms, lose of extraneous body fat will allow you to lose weight, get thinner, stabilize your hormones and reduce or eliminate your PMS symptoms. If you stop walking, this extra glycogen will ultimately be returned to the body and is restored as fat once again. It should be clear that a regular pattern of exercise, vigorous full body upper and lower extremity, walking can assist you in improving your overall health more rapidly and better help you to relive your PMS symptoms.

WHAT KEEPS PEOPLE FROM WALKING?

1. Fear of succeeding.
2. Doing it (exercise) for the wrong reasons.
3. Feeling forced or pushed into it; exercising against your will.
4. Laziness, wanting someone else to exercise for you or making some one else responsible for your participation, "I won't exercise if you don't!"
5. A poor self image, not feeling worthy of reaching your goal.
6. Self anger, hatred or guilt.
7. The need to maintain PMS for protective purposes, to distance some one in your life from you. "I can't be with you this is my PMS week!"
8. Feelings of inadequacy, feeling inadequate to exercise or accomplish goals of wellness and good health.
9. Absence of motivation (all of the above).
10. Lack of a clear picture of what is desired (poor visualization).

For the moment we will simply mention these few reasons, even if they are only a few of the many reasons why people are unwilling or unable to exercise. You may have different reasons specifically related to you and your life situation. If you do talk to some one (a counselor), about these feelings or thoughts.

THERE ARE LEGITIMATE REASONS WHY PEOPLE CANNOT EXERCISE

1. There are chronic conditions such as temporary or even permanent physical or health disabilities, heart disease, amputation, arthritis, problems with feet, knees, ankles, lower or mid back or neck problems, extreme obesity
2. Acute medical problems such as infection, bronchitis, acute strains or sprains of back, legs, feet, ankles or upper extremities, late-term pregnancy to name a few.

Persons with heart disease or other disabilities listed above may require a full evaluation by their physician and either medical clearance or a medically supervised program at a specialized facility.

Individuals with amputations, arthritis, back and neck problems and extreme obesity may or may not be able to exercise depending on the degree of their disability. They may, however, be capable of more than they have tried, with proper preparation and planning, and with gradual conditioning. With the support of their physician, physical therapist or a trainer. they may be able to do more than they previously thought themselves capable of doing.

THERE ARE RELATIVE REASONS WHY PEOPLE CANNOT EXERCISE

- Severe depression, agoraphobia, panic anxiety attacks, chronic fatigue syndrome, fibromyalgia

- No safe area or lack of time to exercise.

Individuals suffering from relative restrictions, may through appropriate treatment of their primary condition, medical or psychological, along with a little creative thought easily be capable of eventually overcoming their problems and form a regular exercise program. If you are not able to perform a standard exercise program, a specialized, tailor-made exercise programs, in some form, can eventually be created for you.

If psychological treatment with or without the use of appropriate medication or problem solving is available, most persons with depression, agoraphobia, panic and anxiety disorders can be ultimately be helped so that they can return to full physical and emotional capacity.

We believe chronic fatigue syndrome to simply be a specific type of depression, one in which the immune and physical systems are involved because of stress or burnout. Exercise along with problem solving and elimination of the triggering problems are often extremely helpful in eliminating this condition. Individuals with fibromyalgia can, with careful help, exercise, even if not strenuously.

THE INTERMEDIATE WALKER

Some readers will possibly already be walking for a while as they make the decision to begin the 30-Days to No More PMS program. Others will soon reach the stage where they are ready for more strenuous and assertive walking. For those of you who are ready and those who will soon be ready there are just a few more points that may be helpful.

1. Before starting your exercising program it is a good idea for you to stretch upper and lower extremity muscles so that you do not get too sore nor end up with spasms or Charlie horses.
2. Set a series of realistic progressive goals so that you can progressively increase your range of exercise to both tone your body and burn unnecessary fat.
3. Remember not to exceed your capacities.
4. Stretch after your walking program.

The advanced walker more than likely needs little or no discussion by us for they are probably already well versed in safety, preparation and stretching.

Whether you are a beginner or intermediate (or even an advanced walker) for specific information about setting up an exercise program, we always suggest working with a professional exercise trainer who can train you and work out a program that will help you accomplish your specific goals. The main advantage of a trainer is that of working with you to show you how to do whatever you wish to do correctly and safely is always of great value. First, and most important of all we remind you that you should not do anything where you can hurt yourself, and secondly, you should only begin what you know you can finish, in order to safely and sanely accomplish your goals.

RUNNING AND JOGGING

Running and jogging requires greater preparation than walking. It is our belief that no one should start to run or jog until they are physically fit, medically checked out and emotionally ready. Both running and jogging can be dangerous and should not be taken lightly or as matter of fact. If you are not already an experienced runner, we strongly recommend taking a class, workshop, personal or group training on how to run. Each year tens of thousands of men and women severely injure themselves because they think that running is simple and easy to do. Running is dangerous if you do not know how to do it correctly, so before you start running make sure you know exactly what you are doing.

Calories Burned During Exercise		
Exercise	Calories/Minute	Calories/Hour
Walking 3 mph	5.2	312
Bicycle riding	8.2	252
Swimming	11.2	672
Running	19.4	1264

The difference between running and jogging is simply a matter of how the feet land on the ground. When an individual runs her foot lands on the ball of the foot, the forward part of the foot. With jogging the foot lands on the heal portion of the foot. This difference may at first sound minimal, however, it is not, for the forces that occur upon your foot landing on the ground effect not only the foot, but also the legs, hip joints, pelvis, low back, middle back, neck and even your head.

Running is a frequent cause of leg and back problems and often causes injuries that not only impair function but can have long term effects on your work and your income as well. Jogging tends to be somewhat safer, that is fewer injuries, but as stated above injuries are still relatively common.

We believe that any person who wants to run or jog should have appropriate foot gear (shoes and stockings), and should have some form of training or at least a consultation by a qualified trainer in the techniques and safety aspects of running or jogging.

The same hints and tips that we gave for walking apply equally for running.

SWIMMING

Once again the same hints and tips apply. If you are a beginning swimmer, make sure that you are up to the task by having some professional instruction in swimming technique before starting any aggressive or strenuous swimming program. In the past we have had patients who begin swimming programs with poor skills, few continue to for very long as they soon tire from the effort that is required when trying to maintain a strenuous program with poor technique. Stretching before and after swimming is also important for safety and injury prevention. Not eating before you swim is also important. Swimming is an excellent cardiovascular exercise and will strengthen your heart and respiratory system. It is good for your whole body.

Swimming is also an excellent form of exercise for toning and conditioning. It is especially valuable for people with back or neck problems, arthritis, problems with the feet or other disabilities as it is a non-weight bearing exercise and will not produce further injury. Swimming can be a valuable exercise as part of a balanced exercise regimen.

Once again, please remember to get a medical check up and professional help in the beginning to support your doing this correctly and safely.

BICYCLING

Bicycling is another excellent sport and a good way to exercise and strengthen your cardiovascular and respiratory systems. The same input is true about bicycling as with walking. You and your bicycle should both be in excellent condition before you start. You should also make have the right clothing and safety devices. Make sure that your seat fits you well and is at the right height for your leg length.

If you wish to perform, advance skills get appropriate training. Never go beyond your capabilities as you increase your chance of injury. Never put yourself in danger. If you ride on the street, on the side of a road your should always be attentive to drivers front and rear. Never ride at night without proper safety equipment, lights or reflectors. If you make long trips such as mountain biking always bring water, and take no chances. Ride in groups and never, if you can help it, alone.

OTHER SPORTS

There are a number of excellent sports that may help you to strengthen your cardiovascular and respiratory systems. For example tennis, golf, volley ball, basketball, soccer, gymnastic and track are all excellent exercise modalities.

Other sports which can be helpful in improving your cardiovascular and respiratory strengthening are football and weight lifting. Both of these sports are however pure power sports, and will often create bulking of muscle and muscle definition. These sports, however, have much higher risk of injury and also relatively short period of ability to play. Once you stop doing these exercises, new muscle tissue will rapidly begin to breakdown and guess what, the breakdown products turn to fat. This is why we see so many fat former football players and former weight lifters. They can produce good muscle toning, change your physique to a more positive look. We do no recommend them for anything but as a weekend sport.

NON-SPORTS ACTIVITIES

Activities such as gardening, dancing, pilates, low impact aerobics, working out at the gym, using home exercising equipment are also valuable. Your ultimate result will depend on how often you do these activities and how strenuous the exercise program is.

Two major advantages are toning and conditioning. They are in themselves extremely valuable and important to overall well-being. If we chose between telling someone to just tone and condition themselves or to exercise to strengthen their cardiovascular and respiratory systems and lose weight we will *always* choose toning and cardiovascular and respiratory conditioning first and weight loss second.

Exercise can also be accomplished by using stairs instead of elevators, parking and walking instead of valet parking. Home units such as stairs steppers and trampolines should only be used with great caution and after training. There are frequent injuries associated with these specific exercises.

Low impact aerobics like walking must be done correctly as injury is possible. The right clothing, proper instruction and building up slowly are all important.

High impact aerobics can be dangerous. You should be accomplished with low impact aerobics, have a capable instructor be in excellent condition and ready for it.

Yoga and Tai-Chi are also excellent all around exercises. They reduce stress, tone and condition, increase muscle bulk and amount of glycogen being used by the muscles. Another value is that they are good general support for release of blocks and complexes. We highly recommend them even if you are doing another more rigorous exercise program.

Meditation, while not usually considered an exercise, can be extremely helpful in toning and reducing stress and releasing blocks and complexes. Therefore, it often supports stress reduction as well as any desired need for managing the anxiety or depression symptoms of PMS. When used along with a active exercise program, as suggested above, they can be even more helpful.

Finally, whichever sport or exercise method you pick you must create a regular routine minimum of at least every three days for it to have lasting affects. Longer than three days means essentially that you are a casual performer and reduces the chance for long-lasting results. Certainly some exercise is better than none at all, however, a regular program is best of all.

WARM UP AND COOL DOWN

No matter which exercise program you decide on, it is essential that you remember to begin your routine by warming up and stretching prior to the vigorous part of the exercise program. There are two main reasons for this 1) prevention of injury, and 2) maximizing the results of your exercise program.

You first want to stretch the major muscle groups to prepare them for your exercise program. This will prevent tearing and muscle injuries. Next you want to begin your program slowly and build slowly until you reach a point where it feels comfortable to begin the strenuous portion of your exercise program. This will allow your heart to reach a place where it can handle strenuous exercise and provides you with maximum heart strengthening. This should take about 5 to 15 minutes of your exercise program.

As you come to the end of your exercise routine allow sufficient time to cool down. This allows your heart rate to return to normal before you have finished your exercise program. The cool down period should also take between 5 and 15 minutes depending on the length of your exercise routine. Once you have finished your program it is also wise to stretch again to relax your muscles before you stop to prevent injury and later muscle spasms.

IN CLOSING

The Metamorphosis 30-Days To No More PMS Dietary Program is an easy, safe, painless and sensible way to reduce or even eliminate your PMS symptoms. By eating the proper foods and adding exercise into your daily routine, you should steadily feel better throughout the duration of the program. We wish for you healthy and happiness and to become fit and trim!

CHAPTER 8

READING LABELS

Throughout our book we have tried to stress over and over again that "What you eat is very important. What you have eaten int the past has caused your PMS and what you eat in the future can eliminate your PMS." We believe that it is most important to eat as much healthy, whole foods as is possible. We generally suggest eating primarily, or even exclusively, certified whole foods. Foods free of insecticides, picked at the end of their growing season and as fresh as is possible. We also have repeatedly stressed that it is important to avoid, as much as is possible refined and processed foods.

However, many people either cannot do this or are unwilling to do this. Often, however, when we are not entirely aware of what we are really eating, especially when eating processed or refined foods. We often select a food based on what we feel like eating or we may choose a food on what we think is good for us. In the past it was often impossible to tell what exactly what ingredients and nutritional components were and were not in the foods we choose to eat unless it was raw and whole. Once a foods are refined or put into a package, we can no longer really be sure of what may or may not be in them. In many cases processed and refined foods have a lot of salt, sugar and often fat, along with other none wholesome substances, are added to them to make them taste better, have a longer shelf life or keep their color and consistency. Often this is done not only to make this food more palatable, but also to addict the user and make her want to eat more than one serving and to select it over all other available foods including more healthy non processed, non refined, whole foods. In the end, this means that these foods are also more profitable, and in many cases profit is the greatest measure of what ends up in or better still out of the food you will ultimately eat.

HOW THEN CAN WE PROTECT OURSELVES?

As long as you continue to purchase and eat packaged, refined and processed foods, it is essential that you learn how to protect your self by learning how to read the labels of every food you purchase so that you know exactly what you are eating, the number of calories, the amount of fat, and the amount of calories from the fat which is in the product. It is also important to know how much saturated and unsaturated fat is present in the product to protect your self from heart disease later in life. It is also important to know whether the product you are purchasing and about to eat contains any unhealthful artificial ingredients such as food dyes, colorings, additives or preservatives. While you may not be able to find all of the information you need to help you with your PMS, you can find a great deal of useful dictary information which can help you in

protecting your overall health while preventing unnecessary weight gain and heart disease simply by reading the nutritional information on the product label. The following suggestions will provide basic information on how to read labels.

1. Start by looking at the front of the package or can. Often the manufacturer will place important information about the product on the front of the package. Often they will make some claims as to the nutritional value and healthfulness of the product. It may say that the product is low in salt or packed in water instead of oil, or in juice instead of syrup. These statements should always be backed up by the "Nutritional Facts" information on the package it self.

2. Next study the "Nutritional Facts" box which is generally located to the right of the front label or on the back of the package. On certain small cans or packages or irregular items it may be located elsewhere or a shortened version may be used. Very small packages may only provide an address or phone number so that you can contact the company for this information.

3. Lastly, look at the ingredient's list. They should we listed in descending order by the amount (weight usually) of the specific ingredient within the product. The place a specific ingredient is located within this list should give you a general idea of the relative amount of that ingredient within the product. Often the specific source of proteins, fats and fiber and some vitamins and minerals may also be listed. Look to see if there are food colorings, dyes, preservatives or additives present. If for example, sugar, corn syrup (see Table 5, below) is listed first this means that the main ingredient in this product, no matter what the label says is in it, is sugar. Remember, foods high in sugar should be avoided is you want to control your PMS.

Sugar Found in Foods in the Following Forms

White table sugar, turbinado sugar, brown sugar, honey, molasses, corn sweetener, corn syrup, any foods which may end in -ose: fructose, dextrose, maltose, dextro-maltose or malto-dextrose, barley sweetener, corn starch and modified food starches, alcohol, white flour, bleached flour, white rice, rice flour, rice vinegar and rice sweetener and processed mashed potatoes.

Table 5

WHAT ELSE SHOULD I KNOW ABOUT THE INFORMATION ON THE LABEL?

1. Since servings sizes vary from product to product, it is often hard to make comparisons without adjusting for serving size. This is easiest done by dividing the serving size into the total amount in the package to find out how many servings are actually in the package. In most cases this is done for you, in others it is not.

2. Most of the information provided is based on a 2,000 calorie-per-day diet. Generally this has no real meaning to the average person unless they are eating a total of 2,000 calories each day. If you are eating 1,200 calories/day or 2,500 calories/day you will have to adjust the numbers up or down. Since most people have no idea exactly how many calories they are eating it is virtually meaningless.

3. No single food contains a full compliment of vitamins, minerals, proteins, fiber and other essential nutrients. Therefore, it is likely that whatever packaged or canned food you are about to use will have to be combined with either fresh foods or other canned or packaged foods to create a totally balanced diet and this generally rarely happens. The total of these foods should be taken into consideration in making any final choices. Your total diet on a day by day basis should be as perfectly balanced as you can make it.

4. Many calorie dense ingredients are disguised so that you will not recognize what they are. For example, sugars are often represented as: sucrose, dextrose, maltose, malt barely, dextrin, malto-dextrin, fructose, honey, turbinado (sugar), brown sugar, molasses, corn sweetener, corn syrup, corn starch and modified food starches. This is a partial list of the way sugars are hidden without having to call them *sugars*. (See Table 5.)

5. When the manufacturer says that the food is low in fat ("Fat Free" or "98% Fat Free) or sugar ("Sugar Free" or "Reduced Sugar") ask yourself as compared to what? Often the amount of fat or sugar (now supposedly reduced) had to be compared to their high fat or high sugar version of the same product. It may not really be low either in fat or sugar. Check the label contents for amount of fat and sugar and also the amount of calories from fat and sugar. You may ultimately have an entirely different picture of what they mean when the manufacturer say, "No" or "Low" fat or sugar and what this really means to them. Hint: "Truth in advertising has always been a lie."

6. Consider the following rule: Products which say that they are, "No Fat," "Low Fat," or have "Reduced Fat," often have increased their total amount of sugar (carbohydrates) added in order to compensate for the reduction in fat content. The same is true when the label reads "No Sugar," "Low Sugar," or "Reduced Sugar," the manufacturer has often added additional fat in order to increase the taste of the food to make it more marketable. When fat or sugar is added to a product it make it taste better and holds up its overall sales. It will only worsen your PMS however. Why do you think you have PMS to begin with?

Nutrition Facts

Serving Size 1 cup (236g)
Servings Per Container about 5

Amount Per Serving

Calories 230 Calories from Fat 120

	% Daily Value *
Total Fat 13 g	**22%**
Saturated Fat 5g	**35%**
Cholesterol 30mg	**13%**
Sodium 118 mg	**5%**
Total Carbohydrates 31g	**5%**
Dietary Fiber 2g	**8%**
Sugars 3g	
Protein 11g	

Vitamin A 20%	•	Vitamin C 0%
Calcium 2%	•	Iron 6%

* Percent Daily Values are based on a 2,000 calorie diet. Your daily values may be higher or lower depending on your calorie needs

	Calories:	2,000	2,500
Total Fat	Less than	65g	80g
Sat Fat	Less than	20g	25g
Cholesterol	Less than	300mg	300mg
Sodium	Less than	2400mg	2400mg

Table 12

READING LABELS:

1. **Nutritional Facts**

This box enables you to quickly determine how much of your daily nutrient requirements will actually be met by eating this specific food.

2. **Serving Sizes**

The servings are meant to standardize the amount of food eaten from item to item and person to person. All the information that follows is based on these amounts. If you eat more or less adjust the nutrient amounts. If you are not aware of the serving size you can over eat the product. For example: If you ate one serving of the product listed in Table 11 you would be getting 230 total calories of which 120 of these calories was from fat. If you were to eat the whole box 5 cups, which in some cases is very easy to do, you would be eating 1,150 calories of which 600 of these calories would becoming from the 65 grams of fat in this product. Becomes an entirely different nutritional experience when you understand it this way.

3. **Calories From Fat**

Knowing the amount of calories created by fat in the specific food can help you to decide which foods to choose. Notice that more than 50% of the calories in this food is from fat. That is, 120 calories of the total 230 calories in this food. Look at it this way $120/230 = \frac{1}{2}$ or one half, hence 50% of the calories. Present recommendations of fat ingestion suggests that fat should make up less than 30% of your daily calories.

That is for optimum health, the percentage of fat in your diet should be *no more* than 30% of the total calories you eat. Ideally for best results no food should contain *no more than* 10% to

20% of its calories from fat in your overall diet.

Also please notice on the label that it is ultimately misleading as it implies that there is only 22% fat in this food, what this really means is that already contains 22% of the fat that is anticipated from a 2000 calorie diet. If you were to eat the entire 5 cups, or 5 times 22%, would mean that this food alone would make up more than 110% of your fat requirement for that day. Everything else you eat during this day which has any fat in it, would simply add to this number and increase your total fat intake for the day above this.

4. **% Daily Value**

This value tells you how much of a nutrient the product provides. We discussed how misleading this part of the Nutritional Facts label can be when we discussed total fat above. Lets look at fiber next. Here one serving of this product supplies 2 grams of dietary fiber which is 8 percent of the recommended daily consumption of 2,000 calorie-per-day diet. The goal is to eat an average of close to 100% of each nutrient daily. If we were to try to do this by eating more of this product we would have to eat nearly 12.5 servings of this food which would mean that you would also be getting more than 12.5 times 22 = 275% of your daily fat from this product. This is a clue that if you are eating one serving of this food you should next chose a series of foods that are higher in fiber and lower in fat.

Listings are also included for of saturated fat, cholesterol, sodium and sugars reflect the need for consumers to either limit or control use these items.

5. **The Lower Three Sections**

These last three sections are only included on larger packages. They show:

1) The inclusion of dietary fiber, calcium, iron and vitamins A and C reflect the need to get adequate amounts of these. Magnesium and B vitamins are omitted from the Nutritional Facts, Table 11 hence you cannot use Nutritional Facts to judge how much of these nutrients are in this product which is no help for controlling your PMS.

2) Daily amounts of certain nutrients required for good health based on both 2,000 and 2,5000 calorie-per-day diets.

3) Calories per gram of fat, carbohydrate and protein. You can use this information when applicable.

6. **Is This Food, a Good Food to Eat?**

Notice that in this example that more than 50% of the calories in this food are from fat. This food also has 31 grams of carbohydrate, 3 grams of which are sugar. We are given no clear indication in the Nutritional Facts section of how many calories this adds until we look down at the very bottom where we see that fat has 9 calories per gram, proteins and carbohydrates have 4 calories per each gram. Nor do we know that these calories are from until we read the list of ingredients.

We can now see that the 31 grams of carbohydrates represent 124 calories (31 rams times 4 calories = 124 total calories). Of this 12 calories (3 times 4) are from sugar. When we add total of the fat calories (120)to the total of the sugar calories (12) we have a totals 132 calories from fat and sugar. This means that a bit more than 57% of the calories in this product are non-nutritive. That is, empty calories, food that has calories but inadequate nutrients. This would be a low-nutritional density food.

Finally, when we evaluate the type of carbohydrate in this product all we know that it this is not a fruit or vegetable, since this food contains such a large amount of fat. It may contain fruits or vegetables but they have been processed, that is cooked and or dehydrated hence many o their nutrients are already removed. We also know that only 2 grams of this food is fiber. Therefore, we are left with 31 grams minus 3 grams of sugar and 3 grams of fiber, a total of 25 grams which is most likely either starch or grain. Since it is more than likely a processed food, it is then more than likely that any grain in it is a processed white flour and hence has little nutritive value. If it is starch, than we have 26 grams (104 calories) more of empty non-nutritive food. This increases the total of non-nutritive food to nearly 95%. This is not likely to be a good food to eat (if health is your goral) as it has a great deal of empty calories.

**Read Labels and Discover
What Is Really
in the Foods You Are Eating.**

CHAPTER 9

Summary of Recommended Treatment for Your Day to Day Use

We have now completed the majority of our 30-Days to No More PMS program. In order for you to get maximum value from it this chapter will be directed as a summary of the dietary program.

1. Most essential is to eliminate as much as possible all dairy products, simple carbohydrates (which includes: white table sugars, brown sugars, turbinado sugars, molasses, honey, alcohol, processed foods, white rice, white flour and foods made with processed fructose) and caffeine foods and beverages, such as coffee, teas, sugary soda pops and chocolate. (See Table 5.)

2. Significantly increase your intake of complex carbohydrates in the form of whole grains, beans, nuts, fruits, yellow, green and red vegetables and cereals that are high in magnesium and vitamin B6. (See basic and Advanced PMS Diets)

3. Next is to limit red meats, animal fats and proteins to no more than 3 ounces daily.(See basic and Advanced PMS Diets)

4. Limit or, better yet, eliminate the use of tobacco, as nicotine reduces useable vitamin B6.

5. Rely more on fish and poultry for your animal proteins. (See basic and Advanced PMS Diets)

6. Use legume and/or grain proteins wherever possible. (See basic and Advanced PMS Diets)

7. Increase foods with cis-Linoleic acid i.e. safflower oil or avocado are an excellent source.

8. Divide what you eat during the day into 4-6 small meals and avoid skipping meals or having single large meals. (See basic and Advanced PMS Diets)

OTHER VALUABLE SUGGESTIONS

1. Exercise at least ½ hour each day. (gardening, swimming, walking briskly at least 4-5 miles

per hour or bicycling.) Avoid strenuous and violent exercise as they can impair liver function and worsen PMS symptoms. Exercise as often as possible outdoors in fresh morning air. Sunlight at this time is best to promote creation of natural vitamin D. Results of indoor exercise are less productive than outdoor exercise. (See Chapter 7, Exercise Is Essential for Treating PMS)

2. Get ample sleep and rest for your needs.

3. Try to schedule stressful events at times other than premenstrually, when possible. Reduce stress in your life whenever possible.

4. Keep a daily diary of your symptoms to help regulate your diet and the amount of supplements you need to be symptom free. (See Personal Management Diary-Daily Symptom Record in the Forms Section in the back of the book.)

5. Each time you take your vitamin-mineral supplements repeat the following affirmation:

> **"I Am Taking an Active Part in**
> **Creating My Own Good Health**
> **and Well Being."**

6. Re-read Chapter 5, Foods to Avoid–Foods To Eat, to be aware of which foods are high in calcium and should be avoided and which foods are high in magnesium and should be included and desired.

7. Read and learn as much as you can about PMS so that you fully understand it. Know what to look for so that you are in complete charge of your body and your life.

TEN OF LISA'S FAVORITE HINTS TO QUICKLY RAISE YOUR MAGNESIUM LEVELS

1. One medium banana will give quick results when you need it.

2. Carry in your purse one ounce of dry roasted unsalted peanuts or raw cashews

3. When you're down try one or two brown-rice or multi-grain cakes. If you want a real pick-me-up, spread a teaspoon of unsweetened peanut butter on each cake.

4. If you're not in the mood for cakes put the peanut butter on celery sticks.

5. Make a trail mix with fruit-juice-sweetened puffed wheat, corn or rice (1 cup) and (1/4 cup) dry roasted unsalted or lightly salted peanuts or cashews. This mixture travels well.

6. Popcorn is one of a number of excellent high magnesium snacks that provides easy, quick opportunities to raise magnesium levels.

7. When you bake or make cereal (dry or cooked) add Ener-G rice bran, corn bran or wheat germ to give you a magnesium boost for the day.

8. Eat ½ medium ripe avocado.

9. Add two Rye Krisp Crackers to the avocado.

10. Put a few slices of banana or a teaspoon of unsweetened peanut butter or both on two Rye Krisp crackers.

The End

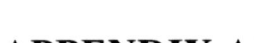
APPENDIX A

TEN WAYS TO ELIMINATE OR REDUCE YOUR PMS SYMPTOMS

PMS affects between 40% and 60% of all women to some extent or another during some time in their reproductive years. Symptoms can range from mild fluid retention all the way to severe mood swings or incapacitating depression.

1. Educate yourself as to what PMS is, what causes it, the lifestyle and dietary measures you can use to prevent or eliminate it.

2. Since PMS is a hormonal imbalance problem created because of a poor diet, one with both excesses of refined and processed foods and deficiencies of magnesium, vitamin B6 a along with other essential nutrients, eating a whole food, nutritionally rich diet and staying away from refined and processed foods, reducing as much as possible your intake of refined sugar and alcohol.

3. Other valuable dietary changes can help reduce the PMS symptoms include the following: a low-fat vegetarian-based diet, reducing as much as is possible the amount of salt, red meats, and caffeine in your diet. Poultry and fish are okay. Increasing your consumption of complex carbohydrates, leafy green vegetables, fruits, cereals and whole grains is generally extremely helpful for most PMS women.

4. One of the best very ways to reduce PMS symptoms is through a regular daily exercise program. Not only does exercise reduce, or sometimes eliminate PMS symptoms, but it is also an excellent way to reduce stress and lower your risks of heart disease, cancer and osteoporosis.

5. Women who experience premenstrual breast tenderness can take 600 IU of Vitamin E daily. In some women vitamin E helps to reduce breast tenderness.

6. Women who find themselves craving sugar during the days when they are experiencing PMS may find relief by supplementing their diet with 300 mg to 800 mg of magnesium daily. Magnesium also may help reduce breast tenderness. Remember to start magnesium slowly and allow your gastrointestinal tract to get use to it.

7. Taking between 50 mg to 300 mg of Vitamin B6 daily will help some PMS women decrease their symptoms. Care should be taken not to overdose on Vitamin B6 as side effects such as numbness can occur when too much vitamin B6 is consumed.

8. An alternative treatment that can be helpful includes taking about 1500 mg of Primrose oil daily, or using natural progesterone cream (amount varies by product).

9. Some women may be able to control their PMS symptoms by using oral contraceptives; however it's important that you weigh the pros and cons of hormonal treatment since there are side effects which can sometimes be more of a problem than their original PMS symptoms.

10. Over-the-counter products such as ibuprofen, naproxen can help to relieve some PMS symptoms, one such product which works for some women is Midol. Aspirin may not be a good choice for women during menstruation because of its potential to increase the length and severity of menstrual bleeding.

APPENDIX B

PLANNING AHEAD FOR ELIMINATING YOUR PMS

PLANNING AHEAD

There six areas of planning ahead that are essential for being successful in eliminating your PMS. They are 1) shopping at the market, 2) meal preparation, 3) eating out, 4) eating on the job, 5) out and about and 6) periods of stress.

Shopping for Food and Food Preparation:

One of the major factors in successfully treating and eliminating your PMS is what you eat and how you shop for it. We have discussed in great detail the goals of eating to eliminate PMS, foods high in magnesium and vitamin B6 and reduction and if possibly elimination of refined and processed foods. The problem is that the nutritional deficiencies and excess we are attempting to reverse often start during childhood with poor eating habits and then continues into adulthood with buying refined and processed foods that are low in nutrition value. During your childhood the problem was created by the types of foods your mother picked for you at the market but as you have grown up and have become responsible for yourself your PMS symptoms have been potentiated by what you have been purchasing at the market and what you are eating when you eat out.

If you do not have foods that potentiate your PMS in your home you will not be eating them and they will no longer be potentiating your PMS. Wise shopping is extremely important. Here are a few tips that can help you a lot in ensuring success in our 30-Days to No More PMS program.

TIPS FOR BEST RESULT WHEN SHOPPING AT THE MARKET

1. Never shop when you are hungry. This will reduce impulse buying.
2. Always have a list of foods you wish to purchase made up in advance before you go shopping. This will also help to reduce impulse buying. Never buy anything that is not on your list unless it is a sundry or household product or you know that it will help you to eliminate your PMS.
3. Whenever you must go to any store which contains food and food products that you may be addicted to, such as bakery goods, sweets, ice cream, candy, chocolate, etc. and you know that you will likely have a problem not buying or sampling them, send a family member to buy what is needed.
4. Ask your family to do without any foods that are particularly a problem for you. This need not be forever for once you have centered yourself and lost your craving for the addictive

Offender Foods, they can once again have their food back.

5. Read Labels (See Chapter 8, Reading Labels) carefully, know what you are buying and eating.
6. Never buy any food that you **know** you will have a problem with.

FOOD PREPARATION

1. Ask others to help out with cooking or shopping when you know that you might have a problem with food preparation.
2. If you can make the same identical anti-PMS foods for everyone in your family.
3. If you cannot make only anti-PMS foods, then before starting to cook drink a full eight ounce glass of water. This will help to fill you up and reduce your chances of "over tasting" foods that might be a problem.
4. Another trick which can also help prevent eating any "Offender Foods" while you are cooking is to chew a stick of sugarless gum. Still do the water first.
5. Do not sample foods that you know you should not be eating. If they do not taste perfectly this will be the price your family pays for not supporting your anti-PMS diet 100%. This is not punitive, simply reality of you having to take care of yourself.
6. Make your anti-PMS foods taste so good that you will not want to cheat and you will enjoy everything you eat.
7. If you are not sure how to do this then buy one or more cook books that will help you make the tastiest foods possible.
8. Use lots of seasonings and spices

EATING OUT

1. Pick restaurants you know will have foods that are on the 30-Days To No More PMS Diet program. If you are not sure reread the Desired Foods Lists and check out the restaurant menu even before you sit down. Today you can often get restaurant menus via the internet. Try this even before you travel to the restaurant.
2. You can always ask for what you want. All you have to do is know what you want to eat and ask for it.
3. Plan ahead. Decide what you want so that when you can order or tell the food server exactly what you want and how to prepare it.
4. Often people are afraid to ask for what they want, so here's a tip if you are one of these people: You are paying for what you get, so get what you want. If your food server is unwilling to bring you what you want and need then, a) get up and leave, b) talk to the restaurant manager, or c) do not patronize that establishment again. If your food server is uncooperative don't leave him or her any tip, tips are for service, if you do not get service then they deserve nothing. This may at fist sound awful but change is only made when people demand more...think of the next woman after you...or what would have happened if the last woman would have demanded a and left without giving a tip...the server would more than likely learn form his or her mistake, hopefully, anyway.

5. Often people on diets feel embarrassed to ask for what they want or to have to hassle with the food server when they have family or business associates at the table with them. There are several things you can do about this. a) You can write out on your business card or a piece of paper exactly what you want, before you go to the restaurant and have it ready to hand to the food server, b) you can call ahead and order, c) you can excuse yourself and talk to the food server, manager or owner away from the table, and d) you can make sure you go to a restaurant where they know you and will give you exactly what you want. "Suzy, I will have my usual."

6. If the restaurant does not have the foods you need bring them with you. Lisa often brings low calories-low fat salad dressing with her when she knows that it is not available.

EATING WHILE ON THE JOB OR TRAVELING

1. At business or social affairs when you order drinks order a Club Soda with a twist of lemon, a diet coke, diet Sprit or herbal ice tea. If anyone give you trouble tell the food server to put a lemon or lime in whatever you are drinking , even water, and it will appear like an alcoholic drink to everyone around you.

2. Do not allow yourself to feel guilty if someone makes a comment when you have celery sticks or Club soda. Ignore them or tell them it is none of their business.

3. When you are invited out to business or social functions call ahead and order what you want and need. You can call the person who is in charge, the Maitre' de, or even the Chief. Tell them that you are on a special diet and you must eat from a particular group of foods. Tell them what you need and expect that you will get it.

4. When traveling on an airline or train call ahead. Tell them you are on a special diet and ask what is available to you. Order whatever you can that is in your best interest. If you cannot get what you need, then bring a healthy high magnesium snack with you to add to your food, or bring extra supplements to balance you out.

5. Bring healthy snacks such as fruits, rice cakes, whole grain bread stick or all you can eat vegetables such as celery, cucumber or zucchini sticks with you. You can have a water, ice tea, broth or soft drinks in a insulated carrier.

6. AVOID VENDING MACHINES. It is rare that they will have anything that is healthy or that will be on your anti-PMS diet.

7. Avoid food, cakes, candies, donuts or other goodies that you should not be eating when they are brought into the office. Learn to say, "No, Thank You!"

8. Don't work around food. If others are eating, and you are tempted, leave.

9. If people are talking about food excuse yourself from the conversation.

WHEN OUT AND ABOUT

1. Our day is not always made up entirely of work, food preparation and dining. There are times we go places such as ball games, movies, card games or other places where food is served. Avoid cookies, cakes, pretzels, candies, hors devours, alcoholic drinks, popcorn with butter, hot dog buns, hamburger on a bun with everything on them, or even some things on them.

2. Take healthy snacks with you to support yourself. See Chapter 9, especially, *Lisa's Favorite Hints to Quickly Raise Your Magnesium Levels.*
3. Don't center any day, event or evening around food, unless you can get the foods you need to have.

SOLUTIONS TO STRESS AND ANXIETY EATING

Stress and hunger often occur about the same time. Sometimes hunger occurs from boredom or hidden anxiety. When this happens you may find yourself eating and not know why. Frequently however, you may recognize what is happening but without having an alternative plan ends up eating. Think ahead and make continency plans, if possible.

This type of eating can be mastered if you are willing to use positive diversions to reduce stress or anxiety and create a more productive way of response to either. In Table 12, we have a list of tried and tested activities that can provide rapid, if not immediate, stress reduction and a diversion away from eating as a habitual response. With time and retraining it is possible to new healthier outlets for old problems.

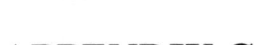

APPENDIX C

VITAMIN B-6

The chemical name of vitamin B_6 is pyridoxine hydrochloride. Other forms of vitamin B_6 include pyridoxal, and pyridoxamine. All three of these compounds are found in the human body. About 70%-80% of the vitamin B_6 in the body is located in muscle bound to glycogen phosphorylase, an enzyme involved in releasing glucose from glycogen. About 10% is located in the liver where it is used to create conjugated estrogen as well as other chemical reactions involving sugar metabolism; the remainder is distributed among the other tissues of the body.

Vitamin B_6 is one of the most versatile enzyme cofactors. It is involved in breaking more types of chemical bonds than almost any other cofactor. It is a component in approximately 120 different enzymes including at least one in 5 of the 6 major enzyme classes. It is involved in the metabolism of amino acids and neurotransmitters and in the breakdown of glycogen into blood sugar. It can bind to steroid hormone receptors and may have a role in regulating steroid hormone action.

Deficiencies: Alterations in the function of the nervous system evidenced by electroencephalography are among the earliest symptoms of vitamin B-6 deficiency. Severe deficiency may produce seizures, dermatitis, glossitis, cheilosis, angular stomatitis and anemia. Frank deficiencies are rare, but subclinical deficiencies may exist, especially in women and the elderly.

DIET RECOMMENDATIONS (RDA'S):

Who	Age Group	Daily Dosage
Children	9-13 years old	1.0 mg daily
Adult Women	14 - 18 yrs	1.2 mg daily
	19-50 yrs	1.3 mg daily
	51+ years	1.5 mg daily
During pregnancy	All ages	1.9 mg daily
During breast feeding	All ages	2.0 mg daily

FOOD SOURCES

White meats (poultry, fish, pork), bananas and whole grains are good sources of vitamin B6.

CLINICAL VALUE

1. Pyridoxine deficiency can cause certain types of seizures and some types of anemias.
2. Vitamin B6 when used with folic acid and vitamin B12 can help to lower plasma homocysteine, a risk factor for heart disease.
3. Vitamin B6 supplements may be required in conjunction with a number of medications which have the side-effect of altering vitamin B6 metabolism.
4. Increased concentrations of pyridoxal phosphate in plasma are used as one of the criteria for diagnosing disorders causing lowered phosphates in the blood .
5. Vitamin B6 metabolism is altered by a variety of disease states, and vitamin B6 supplements may be beneficial in many conditions. PMS is one of these conditions.

FOODS HIGH IN VITAMIN B6

1. Whole grain cereals
2. Sunflower seeds
3. Prunes
4. Liver
5. Filberts
6. Walnuts
7. Potatoes
8. Bananas
9. Turkey and chicken (white meat)
10. Dried apricots
11. Pork and ham
12. Peanuts
13. Peanut butter
14. Sweet potatoes
15. Currants
16. Soybeans
17. Raisins
18. Chicken liver
19. Salmon
20. Tuna
21. Mackerel
22. Lobster
23. Swordfish

OTHER FOODS HIGH IN B6

1. Spinach
2. Bamboo shoots
3. Broccoli, fresh, cooked
4. Vegetable juice, cocktail, canned
5. Sauerkraut, canned
6. Brussels sprouts, frozen, cooked
7. Tomato sauce, canned
8. Carrots, fresh, cooked, juice
9. Zucchini, Italian style, canned
10. Watermelon, raw
11. Potato skin, baked
12. Peas, green, fresh, cooked
13. Yam, Hawaii, steamed
14. Crab, steamed
15. Wheat germ
16. Plantain, cooked
17. Mango, raw
18. Avocado, raw
19. Bulgur, canned

CEREALS

1. Total, Kellogg's
2. Product 19
3. 100% Bran
4. All Bran
5. Bran Buds

APPENDIX D

EAT MORE FRUITS, VEGETABLES, WHOLE GRAINS AND BEANS

Most people know that eating plenty of fruits and vegetables every day is good for your health. However, for the woman with PMS it is almost essential. The National Cancer Institute and the American Heart Association coronary artery and stroke prevention guidelines suggest eating at least 5 or more servings of vegetables and fruit each day. Many people suggest eating even more. Fresh fruits and vegetables not only contain natural sugars (which are good for the body), but they also provide a wealth of essential nutrients the PMS woman must have to undo her already existing vitamin-mineral deficiencies. They can be eaten either raw, such as in salads or fresh fruits, in soups or steamed or even cooked. Grain, as you may well already know is generally high in magnesium and is of vital importance to the woman with PMS. Whole grain breads, cereals or cooked grain as a side dish can quickly undo any magnesium deficiency.

Besides what we have already stated above there are four more reasons to eat more fruits, vegetables and whole grains:

- It is easy to do. They are generally easy to prepare and inexpensive.
- Fruits, vegetables and whole grains are very low in calories, low in fat and have no cholesterol.
- Fruits, vegetables and whole grains are excellent sources of vitamins, minerals, fiber, phytochemicals and other essential and important micronutrients.
- They can help your reduce your risk of heart attack, bowel cancer, macular degeneration and a host of other chronic illnesses.

Here are some simple way you can get started and keep you going in increasing your vegetable and fruits in your diet. Start by try one or two approaches then when you have successfully integrated these try more.

- Buy many kinds of fruits and vegetables when you shop, have plenty of choices, have a variety always on hand so that you never run out of fruits and vegetables.
- Go to a local Farmer's Market to buy certified organic fruits and vegetables whenever you can. These are generally fresher, tastier and have more nutrition as they are picked ripe and sold almost immediately after they are picked. They contain no insecticides, and no synthetic chemicals having been grown in organic fertilizers they are much healthier for you.
- Buy fresh fruits and vegetables in season. Not only will they be cheaper but they also will be at their flavor and nutritional peaks. Always buy vine or tree ripened fruits and vegetables as these are the most nutritious.
- Watch for local specials, fruits and vegetables on sale, if money is an issue.

- When you eat out for lunch try as often as you can to eat at a restaurant which has a salad bar or all you can eat salad and soup restaurant.
- When you eat out for lunch and dinner if you order a salad with you meal and make sure the restaurant uses fresh vegetables only and not canned or cooked with the exception of soups.
- For breakfast try an egg white omelet with a variety of vegetables and the seasonings of your choice.
- As often as you can have a large bowel of soup which is chocked full of high magnesium vegetables (with or without meat in the soup).
- It is okay to occasionally use frozen, dried, or canned vegetables and fruits, however, if you have difficult to control PMS or you are trying to maximize your health allow only fresh fruits and vegetables whenever possible. You can stock up on *fresh flash frozen* vegetables to use in soups and side dishes.
- Always use those fruits and vegetables (for example: peaches, asparagus) that are likely to go bad first.
- Save the hardier varieties (apples, acorn squash) or frozen and canned types for times when you either run out of fresh vegetable or they are not available.
- Take advantage of grocery store salad bars, which offer ready-to-eat raw vegetables and fruits and prepared salads made with fruits and vegetables, especially, if you're in a hurry. This is when you want to make sure that you also have a high magnesium food, such as corn on the cob or whole grain bread as part of your meal.
- Keep a fruit bowl, small packs of applesauce, raisins or other dried fruit on the kitchen counter, table, or in the office. This is much better or you than chocolate or candy.
- Pack a piece of fruit or some cut-up vegetables in your briefcase or backpack; carry moist towelettes for easy cleanup. This will safely prevent episodes of low blood sugar.
- Keep a bowl of cut-up vegetables on the top shelf of the refrigerator. If you are hungry and need to snack use this first instead of junk foods.
- Add fresh fruits or dried raisins to your whole grain breakfast cereal instead of table sugar.
- Add fruits and vegetables to lunch by having them in soup, salad, or cut-up raw instead of any refined food products.
- Add fruits and vegetables to dinner by steaming vegetables and having a special fruit desert.
- Increase portions sizes of vegetables when you serve them. You should be eating 2 to 3 cups of vegetables, fresh, raw steamed or cooked with each meal. Season them the low-fat way with herbs, spices, and lemon juice. If sauce is used, choose a nonfat or low-fat sauce.
- Choose fruit or whole grain bread or cereal for a mid morning snack, for a snack before exercising or for a late night snacks as well as with your breakfast or as a dessert. For a special dessert, try fruit or berries instead of refined sugary products.
- Add extra varieties of high magnesium vegetables when you prepare soups, sauces, and casseroles (for example, corn, mushrooms, potato with skin, avocado (actually a fruit), peas, beets, beans).

THESE IDEAS AND TIPS SHOULD HELP YOU GET STARTED AND THEN KEEP YOU GOING WITH BEANS:

- A few times a week or more, try a low-fat meatless meal or main dish that features beans (along with protein fish or chicken– pinto beans, kidney beans; black beans over a whole grained rice).
- Try canned or frozen kidney beans or black-eyed peas. This can be a fast and easy way to use beans and peas without cooking them from scratch.
- Use beans as a dip for vegetables or filling for sandwiches.
- Serve soup made with beans or peas - minestrone, split-pea, black bean, or lentil (once a week or more). Make your own soup to stay away from processed canned soups loaded with salt, fat or fatty meats.
- Add beans to salads. Many salad bars feature kidney beans, three-bean salad, or chick peas (garbanzo beans).

WHOLE GRAINS ARE EXCELLENT SOURCE OF MAGNESIUM AND VITAMIN B6

- Try whole grin breads.
- Use wild rice, brown rice, millet, whole wheat, barley, buckwheat, rye grain, or Rye Krisp crackers in soups, along with your meal as a side dish, in casserole.
- For breakfast oatmeal is a great trat add raisins or fresh fruit to sweeten it up if you still have a craving for sugary foods.
- Whole grain spaghetti or macaroni (read the label) with a light tomato sauce, lots of mushrooms, low fat hamburger meat can be a tasty high magnesium treat.

DON'T FORGET NUTS AND SEEDS

- Nuts and seeds can be added to bread, casseroles, and other side dishes used as snacks or when you need a sudden infusion of magnesium. Pinyon, pumpkin, ginko, cashew and peanut butter without sugar (add raisins or no-sugar added berry or fruit jams or jelly's to sweeten it up.

REMEMBER THE FOLLOWING:

- All fruits and vegetables should be thoroughly rinsed and washed before eating.
- Wash fruits and vegetables with water and scrub with a brush (never use any soap unless specially made for cleaning vegetables and fruits) when appropriate: for example, before eating apples, cucumbers, potatoes, or other produce in which the outer skin or peeling is consumed.
- Throw away the outer leaves of leafy vegetables, such as lettuce and cabbage.
- Peel and cook when appropriate, although some nutrients and fiber may be lost when produce is peeled.

- Use a salad (glass or plastic) knife to prepare both as this will slow down oxidation (turning brown and decaying) hence they will stay fresh and last longer.
- Variety also is important because fruits and vegetables provide other nutrients, such as folate, potassium, calcium, and iron. Varying choices increases the likelihood of getting all the nutritional advantages of fruits and vegetables.
- Preparation presents another nutritional concern. Since a reduced-fat, reduced-saturated-fat intake is important to a healthful diet, it's important not to overindulge in fruits and vegetables prepared with high-fat ingredients, this includes but is not limited to: meat and vegetable pies, quiche, fried vegetables, such as french fries; cooked vegetables in cheese or cream sauces or with added bacon or butter; fruit pies or fruit served with whipped cream; and dips for raw vegetables. Some of these high-fat foods now have reduced-fat versions, such as low-fat dips and whipped toppings and more often then not they still contain more fat or sugar than you should be eating.
- On all packaged foods read the Nutritional Facts label looking for total fat and total of saturated fats, amount of fiber as well. (See Chapter 8)

TIPS FOR SAFE HANDLING OF FRUITS AND VEGETABLES:

- Wash your hands with warm water and soap for at least 20 seconds before and after handling food, especially fresh whole fruits and vegetables and raw meat, poultry and fish. Clean under fingernails, too.
- Rinse raw produce in warm water. Don't use soap or other detergents. If necessary -- and appropriate -- use a small scrub brush to remove surface dirt.
- Use smooth, durable and nonabsorbent cutting boards that can be cleaned and sanitized easily.
- Wash cutting boards with hot water, soap and a scrub brush to remove food particles. Then sanitize the boards by putting them through the automatic dishwasher or rinsing them in a solution of 1 teaspoon (5 milliliters) of chlorine bleach to 1 quart (about 1 liter) of water. Always wash boards and knives after cutting raw meat, poultry or seafood and before cutting another food to prevent cross-contamination.
- Store cut, peeled and broken-apart fruits and vegetables (such as melon balls) at or below 41 degrees Fahrenheit (5 degrees Celsius) -- that is, in the refrigerator.
- People whose immune systems may be compromised (for example, people who are very young or very old, have a chronic disease, or take certain medicines) should stick with pasteurized juices and cider. Pasteurization kills harmful levels of bacteria commonly found in food.
- When buying from a salad bar, avoid fruits and vegetables that look brownish, slimy or dried out. These are signs that the product has been held at an improper temperature.

Check your Desired Foods List to make Sure you chose high magnesium fruits and vegetables first if you have difficult to control PMS. Once your PMS is under good control, you will not have to do this. When selecting your daily intake of fruits and vegetables, the National Cancer Institute recommends choosing:

- At least one serving of a vitamin A-rich fruit or vegetable a day

30 Days To No More PMS

- At least one serving of a vitamin C-rich fruit or vegetable a day
- At least one serving of a high-fiber fruit or vegetable a day
- Several servings of cruciferous vegetables a week Studies suggest that these vegetables may offer additional protection against certain cancers, although further research is needed.

High in Vitamin A*		
apricots	mustard greens	
cantaloupe	pumpkin	
carrots	romaine lettuce	
kale, collards	spinach	
leaf lettuce	sweet potato	
mango	winter squash (acorn, hubbard)	

High in Vitamin C*		
apricots	grapefruit	plum
broccoli	honeydew melon	potato with skin
brussels sprouts	kiwi fruit	spinach
cabbage	mango	strawberries
cantaloupe	mustard greens	bell peppers
cauliflower	orange	tangerine
chili peppers	orange juice	tomatoes
collards	pineapple	watermelon

High in Fiber or Good Source of Fiber*		
apple	cooked beans and peas (kidney,	orange
banana	navy, lima, and pinto beans,	pear
blackberries	lentils, black-eyed peas)	prunes
blueberries	dates	raspberries
brussels sprouts	figs	spinach
carrots	grapefruit	strawberries
cherries	kiwi fruit	sweet potato

Cruciferous Vegetables
bok choy
broccoli
brussels sprouts
cabbage
cauliflower
leafy green vegetables, spinach, greens of all type

APPENDIX E

CAFFEINE CONTENT OF COMMON FOODS

CAFFEINE IN FOOD, DRINKS, DRUGS

Caffeine is a widely used drug that has been around for centuries. It is a drug. A natural drug but still a drug. It is a naturally occurring substance in coffee beans, cocoa beans, kola nuts and tea leaves which are used to make coffee, tea, cola drinks and chocolate. It is an additive in many soft drinks and nonprescription medications. It does not occur in foods unless coffee beans (coffee), cocoa beans (chocolate), kola nuts (cola drinks) and tea leaves (tea). Caffeine is added to a few medications as a stimulant to energize or to create a sense of increased well-being. Caffeine does not occur naturally in the majority of the other foods a PMS woman would eat or drink.

Coffee is the primary source of caffeine for most Americans, cola drinks and tea follow right behind. Americans consume half of the world's coffee, or more than one thousand cups per person per year. Small to moderate amounts (50-300 mg) of caffeine act as a mild stimulant by increasing the heart rate and blood pressure. However, caffeine is a double-edged sword in that while it provides an initial boost of energy, it not usually sustain this energy boost throughout the day. To maintain the high that it creates you have to drink or ingest more caffeine, if you do not fatigue and withdrawal symptoms will soon come forcing the average person to "need another cup of coffee." or whatever they were using to regain their caffeine high.

Women who ingest excessive amounts of caffeine and those women who are hypersensitive to caffeine, may find themselves experiencing symptoms of an overdose of caffeine: anxiety, trembling, insomnia, headaches, stomach irritations, diarrhea and possibly even an irregular heartbeat. For women, caffeine may also play a role in a number of perplexing problems:

- As you already know it can contribute to risk of PMS
- Fibrocystic breast changes, caffeine is presently being looked at to determine if it plays any role in breast cancer.
- Infertility
- Miscarriage
- Osteoporosis
- Caffeine can aggravate or trigger migraine headaches and might also be associated with chronic back pain.
- Some women experience urinary incontinence as they age. Although caffeine does not cause this condition, women with this condition may experience a greater degree of "urgency" for a short time after consuming a caffeinated beverage.

Studies have also linked caffeine to increased risks of cancer, high blood pressure, heart disease and fibrocystic breast disease. However, most of these claims are still not yet conclusively proven.

Caffeine does appear to clearly aggravate fibrocystic breast disease - but it does not cause it. Fibrocystic breast disease is a condition with benign fibrous lumps in the breast.

CAFFEINE AND FOOD

Caffeine will mask hunger and fatigue and this can lead to poor eating or sleeping habits. It is not unusual for caffeine to be used to provide extra energy when lacking sleep or food. However, ultimately it has been shown to have negative impact on judgment, acuity and physical well-being and lead to sleep deprivation. Continually using caffeine as a means to reducing hunger and avoiding eating in now taken as an early sign of an eating disorder.

MODERATION IS BEST

A moderate amount of caffeine per day, 300 milligrams, or less appears to be relatively harmless for most women.

WHO SHOULD AVOID OR SEVERELY LIMIT CAFFEINE?

Women with ulcers or who are prone to stomach stress Women who are hypersensitive to caffeine. Pregnant and nursing mothers, women with PMS. If you are anemic, be aware that tea and coffee contain substances which can significantly reduce iron absorption if taken during a meal or up to one hour after the meal.

IF MY DAILY INTAKE OF CAFFEINE IS ALREADY HIGH, HOW CAN I REDUCE THE CAFFEINE IN MY DIET?

1. Drink decaffeinated coffee or mix it half and half with regular coffee.
2. Drink decaffeinated tea or caffeine free herbal teas.
3. Brew tea for shorter amounts of time.
4. Avoid citrus flavored sodas as many have more caffeine than colas.
5. One dose of over-the-counter medications can contain the equivalent of one to two cups of coffee.
6. *Read all food and medication labels to see if caffeine is an ingredient and then avoid this medication or food if caffeine is a major ingredient.*

AVERAGE VALUES OF CAFFEINE CONTENT (MG/SERVING)

The list below shows some of the more common products which contain caffeine (it dos not list all products manufactured in the US or in the world), you may consume some of these products along with your daily food intake. Along with the food product we have listed the approximate amount of Caffeine in each serving. Please note that there can be fluctuations due to beans, leaves or coca and brew strength, manufacturing batches, where the product is manufactures and the formulation at the time of the manufacture. Because of ths the values listed in any serving of a specific beverage may vary from product to product and time to time. Also some companies list the value as a 5 oz cup or as 6 oz cup rather than as an 8 oz cup. To know exactly what is in each product you chose to use please read the label and pay attention to the serving size as in some products there may be more than one serving per bottle or package.

Average Values of Caffeine Content	
Food-Drink Product	**mg/unit**
Coffee Beverages, mg/cup (8 oz) or tsp or tablespoon	
Hills Brothers	189 /cup
Dripolated	146 (range 137-153)
Percolated	110 (range 97-125)
Brewed, ground	135 (range 85-200) /tsp
General Foods International Coffee, Orange Cappuccino	102 /cup
General Foods International Coffee, Café Vienna	90 /cup
Starbucks Coffee Frappuccino	83 /cup
Maxwell House Cappuccino, Mocha	60-65 /cup
Maxim, freeze-dried	61 /tsp
Instant Coffee	60 /tsp
Nescafe, Nestle	59 /tsp
Tasters Choice, Nestle	59 /tsp
Mellow Roast (coffee & grain)	56 /cup
Yuban	56 /cup
General Foods International Coffee, Swiss Mocha	55 /tsp
Maxwell House Cappuccino, French Vanilla or Irish Cream	45-50 /tsp
Orange Cappuccino	33 /tsp
Café Vienna	32 /tsp
Café Francais	30 /tsp
Suisse Mocha	29 /tsp
General Foods International Coffee, Viennese Chocolate Café	26 /tsp
Maxwell House Cappuccino, Amaretto	25-30 /tsp
Instant, dccaffeinated	3-5 /tsp
Brim, freeze-dried decaf.	3 /tsp
Sanka	3 /tsp

Sanka, freeze-dried, decaf	3 /tsp
Tasters Choice, decaf, Nestle	5 /tsp
Cocoa/Hot Chocolate Beverages	
Chocolate (1 oz) dark	20 /serving
Chocolate (1 oz) Baker's Chocolate	26 /serving
Cocoa mix, instant	9 /tablespoon
Chocolate (1 oz) milk	6 /serving
Nestle Carnation Rich Chocolate Flavor Hot Cocoa Mix	2 /package
Instant Breakfast, Carnation	trace /package
Instant Brkfst, Choc, Carnation	trace /package
Milkshake, Choc Malt, Delmark	trace /oz.
Tea Beverages / cup	
Celestial Seasonings Iced Lemon Ginseng Tea (16 oz)	100
Bigelow Raspberry Royale Tea	83
Tender Leaf	66
MJB	62
Jacksons of Piccadilly Earl Gray	61
Tetley	61
Twinings English	61
White Rose	61
Teas, brewed from 1 tea bag of most imported brands of brewed black, green or oolong tea	25-110 Average 60
Teas, brewed from 1 tea bag of major U.S. brands of brewed black, green or oolong tea	20-90, Average 40
Our Own	60
Salada	59
Brooke Bond Red Rose	54
Canterbury	54
Lipton, bagged	54
Stewarts	53
Lipton, loose	51
Snapple Iced Tea (16 oz)	48
Grand Union	48
Swee-touch-nee	47
Harvest Day	45

Pantry Pride	45
Royal Jewel	44
Nestle, instant iced w/ lemon	42
Lipton's Iced Teas Assorted (16 oz)	18-40
Nestea Iced Tea (16 oz)	34
Bigelow Constant Comment	31
Bigelow Constant Comment	31
Tea, green	30
Arizona Iced Tea, assorted varieties	15-30
Lipton Soothing Moments Blackberry	25
Nestea Pure Lemon Sweetened Iced Tea	22
Snapple Lemon Iced Tea	19
Tea, instant	15
Lipton Natural Brew Iced Tea Mix, diet	10-15
Nestea Iced Tea Sweetened Lemon	10
Boston's 99 ½% Caffeine-Free	9
Carbonated Beverages mg / 12 oz. (Unless otherwise specified)	
Cola Beverages Per 12 oz.	47 (range 30-90)
Mr. Pibb	57
Mountain Dew	37- 55
Mello Yellow	53
Surge	51
Regular Coca-Cola and Diet Coca-Cola	47
Tab, sugar free	47
Shasta Cola, Cherry Cola and Diet Cola	44
Sunkist Orange Soda (12 oz)	40
Dr. Pepper	41
Dr. Pepper, sugar free	41
Pepsi Cola	27-38
Diet Pepsi Cola	36
Pepsi Light	36
Royal Crown Cola, Diet RC, Diet Rite Cola	36
Coca-Cola	35
Royal Crown Cola, sugar free	33
Canada Dry Cola	30

Pepsi Blue Berry Cola Fusion	26
Coca-Cola Classic	24
Barq's Root Beer	23
Royal Crown Cola w/ a twist	21
Vanilla Coke	21
Barq's Famous Olde Tyme Root Beer	15
Canada Dry Diet Cola	1.2
Mug Root Beer	0
Sprite or Diet Sprite	0
Energy Drinks / 12 oz. (Unless otherwise specified)	
Ripped Force (per serving)	120
AMP Energy Drink	77
Jolt	71
Red Bull Energy Drink	70
Red Fusion	38
Misc. Drinks / 12 oz. (Unless otherwise specified)	
Elements Atomic Jacked Apple Juice Drink	33
dnL	27
SoBee Energy Citrus Flavored Beverage	25
Caffeinated Waters / 12 oz. (Unless otherwise specified)	
Java Water	125
Krank 20	100
Aqua Blast	90
Water Joe	60-70
Aqua Java	50-60
Foods	
Ben & Jerry's No Fat Coffee Fudge Frozen Yogurt (1 cup)	85 /serving
Starbuck's Coffee Ice Cream (1 cup)	40-60 /serving
Dannon Coffee Yogurt (1 cup)	45 /serving
Dark chocolate, 1.5 oz.	100 /serving
Chocolate, milk, 1.5 oz	10-31 /serving
Hershey's Special Dark Chocolate Bar	31 /serving
Perugina Milk Chocolate Bar with Cappuccino Filling	24 /serving
Hershey Bar (milk chocolate)	10 /serving
Coffee Nips (hard candy)	6 /serving

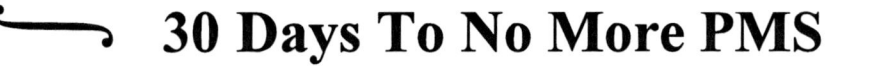

Frozen Desserts	
Ben & Jerry's No Fat Coffee Fudge Frozen Yogurt	85 /serving
Starbucks Coffee Ice Cream, assorted flavors	40-60 /serving
Häagen-Dazs Coffee Ice Cream	58 /serving
Häagen-Dazs Coffee Frozen Yogurt, fat-free	40 /serving
Häagen-Dazs Coffee Fudge Ice Cream, low-fat	30 /serving
Starbucks Frappuccino Bar	15 /serving
Healthy Choice Cappuccino Chocolate Chunk or Cappuccino	8 /serving
Yogurts	
Dannon Coffee Yogurt	45 /serving
Yoplait Café Au Lait Yogurt	5 /serving
Dannon Light Cappuccino Yogurt	< 1 /serving
Drugs (mg/pill)	
Diuretics	167 /tablet
Weight Control aids	150-300
No Doz, Vivarin	100 /tablet
Pre-Mens	66 /tablet
Excedrin, Anacin	64 /tablet
Aspirin compound - Phenacetin-Caffeine (APC)	32 /tablet
Cope, Midol, etc.	32 /tablet
Dristan, Sinarest	30 /tablet

APPENDIX F

MANGANESE AND ZINC

MANGANESE

Manganese helps to control blood sugar levels and with sugar metabolism, improves bone strength and may help in the healing of wounds. Women who smoke are at higher risk for osteoporosis, so they should take some manganese regularly. The usual recommended dosage of manganese in non-pregnant adults range from 150- 30 mg daily.

SYMPTOMS OF DEFICIENCY SYNDROME FOR MANGANESE

Symptoms from manganese deficiency are generally rare, however when they occur they can include: atherosclerosis, elevated cholesterol levels, confusion, tremors, impaired vision and hearing, skin rash, irritability, increased blood pressure, pancreatic damage, impaired sugar metabolism, sweating, increased heart rate, mental impairment, grinding of the teeth.

SOURCES OF MANGANESE

Canned pineapple juice, wheat bran, wheat germ, whole grains, cereals, black beans, oatmeal, seeds, nuts, spinach, strawberries, cocoa, ginger, shellfish, tea, dairy products, apples, apricots, avocados, bananas, Brewers yeast, cantaloupe, grapefruit, green leafy vegetables, peaches, figs, salmon, soybeans, tofu.

ABSORPTION AND TOXICITY OF MANGANESE

Absorption of manganese can be improved when taken with calcium, iron, vitamin B complex, vitamin E.

Generally considered to not be toxic. However, exposure to industrially inhaled manganese has been associated with psychiatric and neurologic disorders.

ZINC

Zinc is essential to the regulation of blood sugar and therefore controls the nutrition of the brain and other organs.

Zinc has a low toxicity in humans, The National Academy of Science however, warns against zinc supplements of more than 15 mg daily without medical supervision except during pregnancy where 20 mg is considered okay. Regular ingestion of more than 50 mg of zinc on a daily basis can however, lead to interference with the absorption of other nutrients and end up causing secondary deficiencies of these nutrients. Copper absorption into the body can be decreased when excessive zinc is ingested on a daily basis. Zinc absorption can be increased when taken with white bread, milk or soy but will be reduced by the presence of bran.

FOOD SOURCES OF ZINC

Zinc rich foods: lean meats (especially beef and lamb), eggs, lentils, beans, lima beans, whole grains and whole grain cereals, oysters, nuts (especially pecans), yogurt, fish, sardines, liver, mushrooms, pumpkin and sunflower seeds, soybeans and poultry.

ZINC SUPPLEMENTS

A large amounts of folic acid can block the intestinal absorption of zinc, thereby creating a potentially dangerous zinc deficiency. To avoid this problem, you should limit your intake of folic acid to no more than 800 mg a day. If you are taking a 800 mg or more of folic acid daily it is advisable to take a little extra zinc. A couple of zinc lozenges of 13 mg/each 2x a day, plus the 20 mg. in your prenatal supplement will give you a potential total of 46 mg in a day. This seems like a relatively safe practice for women getting more than 800 mg of folic acid daily. If you have questions about this discuss it with your doctor to be sure.

ABSORPTION AND TOXICITY OF ZINC

Absorption is improved when zinc is taken with foods or supplement containing calcium, phosphorous, and vitamin B6 (pyridoxine).

Zinc toxicity can create nausea, vomiting, abdominal pain, impaired coordination and fatigue.

Regular ingestion of more than 50 mg of zinc daily can create interference with the absorption of other nutrients, causing secondary deficiencies. Copper is one such mineral whose absorption is depressed with too much zinc. Do not take more than 50 mg of zinc in any one day.

PMS Forms For Personal Use and
To Give To Friends

The following forms and more can be downloaded for free from our website

www.30DaysToNoMorePMS.com

Look for PMS Forms.

30 Days To No More PMS

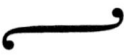

10 MOST FREQUENT FOODS YOU EAT FORM

1. _____

2. _____

3. _____

4. _____

5. _____

6. _____

7. _____

8. _____

9. _____

10. _____

Comments:

_____

_____

_____

_____

_____

_____

_____

_____

_____

_____

PMS Evaluation Questionnaire (PEQ)

Name_____ Date_____ Last Menstrual Period ____/____/_____

Grade Your Symptoms For Your Menstrual Cycle

Symptoms	A Week Before Period	B Week During Period	C Week After Period	
Nervous Tension				**Total from**
Mood Swings				**Week Before**
Irritability				**Scores**
Anxiety				**(Column A)**
	Total	Total	Total	
Weight Gain				**Subtract (—)**
Swelling of				**Total from**
Breast Tenderness				**Week After**
Abdominal Bloating				**Scores**
	Total	Total	Total	**(Column C)**
Headache				
Craving for Sweets				
Increased Appetite				**Equals (=)**
Heart Pounding				
Fatigue				
Dizziness or Fainting				
	Total	Total	Total	**The Severity of Your PMS Symptoms**
Depression				
Forgetfulness				
Crying				
Confusion				
Insomnia				
	Total	Total	Total	

Add All Above for Total Your [____] **Col B** [____] **Col C** [____]

One Week Sample Menu

	Sunday	Monday	Tuesday	Wednesday	Thursday	Friday	Saturday
Breakfast							
AM Snack							
Lunch							
Afternoon Snack							
Dinner							
PM Snack							

Personal Management Diary - Daily Symptoms Record

Name:_____ First Day Last Period ____/___/_____

Grading of Menses (Menstrual Flow)	0-none	3-heavy
	1-slight	4-heavy and clots
	2-moderate	

Grading of Symptoms (Complaints)	
0-none	3-severe
1-mild	4-disabling
2-moderate	

Day of Cycle	1	2	3	4	5	6	7	8	9	10	11	12	13	14	15	16	17	18	19	20	21	22	23	24	25	26	27	28	29	30	31	32	33	34	35
Date																																			
Menstrual Flow																																			

PMS-A Anxiety Group

Nervous tension																																			
Mood Swings																																			
Irritability																																			
Anxiety																																			

PMS-C Cravings Group

Headache																																			
Craving for sweets																																			
Increased appetite																																			
Heat pounding																																			
Fatigue																																			
Dizziness/faintness																																			

PMS-D Depression Group

Depression																																			
Forgetfulness																																			
Crying																																			
Confusion																																			
Insomnia																																			

PMS-H Hydrous Group

Weight gain																																			
Swelling extremities																																			
Breast tenderness																																			
Abdominal Bloating																																			

Dysmenorrhea - Painful Menstruation

Cramps, Low Abdominal																																			
Backache																																			
General																																			

Other Symptoms

Weight

Weight in lbs.																																			

Vitamins-Medications

Vitamins																																			
Medications																																			

Comments:_____

(This Page Is Purposefully Left Blank For You To Use To Take Notes)

CPSIA information can be obtained at www.ICGtesting.com
Printed in the USA
LVOW09s1941050115

421585LV00032B/2212/P